the AGING PROPOSITION

Take Care of Your Body and Mind and Live Youthfully After Age 50

SCOTT ABEL

Edited by Perry Mykleby

Published by:

Scott Abel

© Copyright Scott Abel

ISBN-13: 978-1542903271
ISBN-10: 1542903270

ALL RIGHTS RESERVED. No part of this publication may be reproduced or transmitted in any form whatsoever, electronic, or mechanical, including photocopying, recording, or by any informational storage or retrieval system without express written, dated and signed permission from the author.

Disclaimer

Please consult your family physician or healthcare provider before beginning any new exercise or training program.

The information provided in this book is intended as a resource, and is not to be used or relied upon as medical advice, or as a substitute for medical advice. The information provided in this book is to be used at the sole discretion and risk of the reader.

Table of Contents

Introduction 7

Chapter 1. Fear of Aging 27
Chapter 2. Biological Age, Chronological Age and Psychological Age ... 33
Chapter 3. A New Kind of Youthfulness 47
Chapter 4. Mind-Body and Body-Mind Connection 53
Chapter 5. The Importance of Awareness 83
Chapter 6. Insight, Intuition, Introspection, and the Benefits of Solitude. 101
Chapter 7. Food Matters 119
Chapter 8. Weight Loss and Exercise After 50 137

Conclusion 163
Final Thoughts 177

Appendix 181
A Free Gift 191
Endnotes 197

Introduction

My father lived in a lot of pain near the end of his life. His 70 years of heavy smoking left him with congestive heart failure and it led to open sores all over his legs and feet. This left him wheelchair bound. When he got into the long-term care nursing home he said to me one day, "This is just a place to wait around to die." He passed away three weeks later.

The blunt truth for so many people is that elder years offer an escape from an unfulfilling life. But it doesn't have to be that way. Your fifties are the infancy of your elder years. How you choose to live those years can play a huge role in how the next decades will play out for you. I am going to advise you on how you can put your best foot forward into your future and live a grander life after 50.

This book is about embracing your own aging process. It's about keeping accelerated, premature aging at bay, choosing to see your fifties and sixties as the youth of your elder years.

It is also about understanding and embracing a new kind of youthfulness and how to age fantastically, and be fantastic as you age—"age-tastic"—and what that means mentally, emotionally, physically, behaviorally and even spiritually.

I'd like to begin with a poem called "Youth," from American writer and poet Samuel Ullman (1840-1924). Ullman's piece on youth and youthfulness fits perfectly as an introduction.

"Youth"

Youth is not a time of life; it is a state of mind; it is not a matter of rosy cheeks, red lips and supple knees; it is a matter of the will, a quality of the imagination, a vigor of the emotions; it is the freshness of the deep springs of life.

Youth means a temperamental predominance of courage over timidity of the appetite, for adventure over the love of ease. This often exists in a man of sixty more than a boy of twenty. Nobody grows old merely by a number of years. We grow old by deserting our ideals.

Years may wrinkle the skin, but to give up enthusiasm wrinkles the soul. Worry, fear, self-distrust bows the heart and turns the spirit back to dust.

Whether sixty or sixteen, there is in every human being's heart the lure of wonder, the unfailing child-like appetite of what's next, and the joy of the game of living. In the center of your heart and my heart there is a wireless station; so long as it receives messages of beauty, hope, cheer, courage and power from men and from the infinite, so long are you young.

When the aerials are down, and your spirit is covered with snows of cynicism and the ice of pessimism, then you are grown old, even at twenty, but as long as your aerials are up, to catch the waves of optimism, there is hope you may die young at eighty.

Ask yourself these questions:

1. Are you middle-aged, or age-tastic?
2. Are you over the hill, or climbing mountains?
3. Are you long in the tooth, or young at heart?
4. Are your best years behind you, or right now and ahead of you?

Your answers represent your outlook on aging.

Which ones do you identify with most, not just in your thoughts, but in your day to day behaviors and habits?

When it comes to adulthood, the story line I've read about a thousand times goes something like this: you spend your twenties indulging yourself and trying to figure out what you want. You spend your thirties going after whatever that ends up being. At some point in your forties you "wake up" and ask yourself, *"Is this all there is?"*

And yet, on the flip side, is the old expression,

"Life begins at forty."

But does it? What about after those years? The fact that there is scant attention paid to the fifth decade of life and what it can mean speaks volumes to how little this time of life is valued in our current zeitgeist. But it doesn't have to be that way for you.

Chronologically, I am "middle-aged," and that's fine. The term "middle-aged" does not define me in any way. I am indeed aware of some certain diminished physiological capacities as a result of my body aging. But I don't feel old. In fact, I'm not even sure what the term "feeling old" is even supposed to mean. I am just me, always being me. I have learned a lot at this age. I wouldn't exchange a younger body or more youthful appearance for the wisdom I've gained and the life I get to live right now.

I am very fortunate. I stumbled on an avocation in my younger years that became a career for me. It just happened to be a career in fitness and physique development that leads to a great lifestyle, a lifestyle that brings benefits to any age person. But my passion for exercise and physique development has expanded into other elements of overall health, wellness and well-being. I now find myself in a lifestyle of youthfulness: how to stay young metaphorically and spiritually while growing older chronologically. I'd like to share these insights with you in this book.

I first wrote the book *Physique After 50* to discuss the best forms of exercise for us as we age. That book was a solid first step. However, there are other quality-of-life issues to cover about living in an aging body; and I didn't want to leave a trite impression that having a better physique after age 50 should be the ultimate goal.

Several insights occurred to me about this during my summer vacation. I was stopped several times during those weeks by people asking my age. Most comments were along the lines of "Wow, you look fantastic." Or, "No way I would have guessed you are 55 years old." We were at Starbucks one morning getting our caffeine fix when a man approached me and said, "Pardon me for interrupting but I noticed you as soon as you came in and I just had to come over and talk with you." He was very enthused about my physique and my age in comparison. This man was also in his fifties. He said he follows an older Youtube exercise guru who I had never heard of, then went on to say that I look way better than him, and said that he would follow me in a heartbeat if I did something similar. He asked me about my training and my diet, and said just seeing me inspired him. I was quite flattered and gave him my website address. It gave me a feeling of satisfaction, given that I had only recently finished *Physique After 50*.

I got comments and questions like that throughout my vacation. It reminded me of my former professional physique days when I would sign autographs and take pictures with fans. But I am hardly that caricature of an over-developed physique specimen anymore. Another night at dinner, a waiter came by and asked permission for one of the bus-boys to come by the table and meet me. I agreed of course. The lad of probably no more than 23 years old recognized me because he follows me online, and told me he just had to meet me. Once again I was flattered.

Beyond all of this flattery was a deeper meaning for me. I thought about how many 55-year-olds are engaged by strangers because they want to share how great they look, or ask about diet and exercise. It occurred to me how incomplete all of these superficial observations actually are. If I look great, it's because I live great. It's because my self-directed thoughts lead to my day to day habits, regimens and lifestyle behaviors that manifest themselves in an impressive appearance. It's certainly not some kind of secret. The most important things in my life now boil down to two words: satisfaction and contentment. I created the term "age-tastic" to describe the kind of youthfulness and vigor in aging that I am attempting to impart here.

After contemplating all of this, I had to write this sequel to *Physique After 50* to go beyond the realm of physical fitness and discuss how to be age-tastic. So let's get to it.

* * *

You can't just lump people together in one single demographic and then predict their life experience. Aging is like that. It is the individual, not the age that matters.

The things that hamper us as we age are not so much about the years, but all the potential ills and limitations that seem to come with those years. Plato said, "Fear old age, for it does not come alone." But a lot has changed since Plato's time. Health care and technology are better. We lead lives of ease, convenience, and abundance. These have perhaps contributed to a better aging experience.

Maybe we don't have to "fear old age" as Plato put it. Your fifties and sixties can be the youth of your later years if you make them that way and don't passively accept your age. Becoming age-tastic isn't about bullet-proofing yourself against aging. That simply isn't possible. Being age-tastic is about living a lifestyle of wellness, controlling the things you can in order to age better. Your body will gradually deteriorate away from optimal function. This begins happening sooner than we realize, but we don't have to invite aging or think we are helpless to do anything about it. And we certainly don't have to invite premature or accelerated aging. Yet so many of you do exactly that by the way you think, and the way you live your lives.

Here is something to ponder. Do you remember when you were a kid of age eight to 10, and what you considered "old?" When you were that age, did you ever imagine what you would be like at age 50? Very likely you did not, and if you did, it was very likely much different from the reality of living it. Now that you are an adult, you may want to ponder doing this exercise again for real from the vantage point of a more mature and experienced mind. You may be in your fifties now, as I am, but with modern medicine and technology you may live another 40 years or more; basically another half of your life. So how is this going to play out for you? How do you see yourself at age 85, maybe age 90? What are you going to do, or not do, to make this vision happen? This becomes your "aging proposition."

I want you to visualize the next 30 to 40 years that lie ahead of you. If you continue living your current lifestyle, what do you see for yourself? What is your life's trajectory? Is this a positive or negative proposition for you? What are you willing to do about it starting right now?

Our generation is lucky: it doesn't get set out to pasture as if we are too old to work and contribute. You can retire and still be productive. You can pursue other interests. You don't have to just sit in a rocking chair and let age happen to you. You are likely shaped, molded and more realistic by life experience. I know I am. Hopefully your mid-life crisis, seven year itch, and all those other clichés years are behind you. So, what do you see for yourself? Are you merely alive, or are you still living your life?

You know that if you're 50 or older, that things are different for you physically than they were in your younger years. These years are different. You can no longer just wistfully assign something you want to do to the notion of "someday."

Set aside the stereotypes of aging and your worries about Alzheimer's, dementia, cardiovascular disease and the other haunting scenarios that may exist in your vision of your own aging. Plato's quote notwithstanding, there is a difference between "aging" and "being old." What do you want for yourself and for your life for these next 30 or 40 years? Do these wants invigorate you, scare you, or depress you? What are you now willing to do to set it in motion or improve the visualization you've just created? Everything you think and feel in relation to these things; this is who you are; and who you are being. So when it comes to "age" being something that is happening to you; what do your thoughts and feelings about this tell you about who you really are? And if that is too deep a question for you then you should probably stop reading this project right now.

With modern medicine, you are likely going to be old for a very long time. Think about that for a minute and let it reverberate. How do you want those years to be for you? Let's consider some very pertinent context about all this shall we; I hope the following will give you some very relevant perspective. I know it certainly has for me. So here goes:

Around the time of the Roman Empire, life expectancy was a mere 28 years. Most people died before age 30! Before the turn of the twentieth century, only one in ten people even lived to age 65. In 1900, the average US lifespan was 49 years. However, by the 2014 census, this lifespan has almost doubled to 78.7 years. This means that since the early 1900s, life expectancy has increased by more than 50 percent.

Medicine and technology has given a gift of longer life. We should be responsible and appreciative of that gift and aim for a higher quality of life with the extra years. While only 10 percent of the population once make it to age 65, now greater than 80 percent of the population does. You get to decide how to live those extra years.

I now run into so many people I used to know—once alive and brimming with goals and ideas—who almost seem to have given up. They are often dull, cynical, with a tiny, narrow world view. Their ambitions have shrunk and their bodies have expanded. They seem to have allowed their minds to grow old and their bodies just followed that lead.

Make no mistake what I am saying here. There is a big difference between acceptance of aging and just general dispirited indifference to aging, and by extension, to life itself. That's a big and bold one-sided statement I know, but I witness this week in and week out.

For example, I got an email recently from John V.

Apparently we went to high school together. He was researching dieting and weight loss online and ended up on my website.

Then he wrote me his story:

> Scott,
>
> I can't believe I accidentally found you online. I've been looking for someone to help me and I didn't even know you were in the fitness field. I hope you remember me. We went to high school together although we hung in different crowds and I was a year or two behind you. That seems so long ago, doesn't it? I really need help. I have gained some weight and I have some serious health issues. I've been divorced twice and neither one has been amicable. I pay alimony to

two wives and I have 2 kids from each marriage. I feel like with work and all these other obligations I have lost myself as well. I have depression and anxiety and I take meds for these conditions as well as strong medication for sleep as well. But now I kind of feel like a zombie most of the time. I smoke about a pack a day of cigarettes but I'd like to quit. I want my life back. I want to get healthy again. I know I need to make the time for this but I never seem to have the time. It seems like an excuse but I also don't seem to have the energy either. I just turned 53 years old and I feel like my life is passing me by.

Can you help me?

John's letter above doesn't paint a very good picture for aging well. He's only just 53 but he's already feeling old. A lot of this has to do with earlier lifestyle choices, either for self-indulgence or to deal with stress. Lifestyles are difficult things to change, no question about it. For John, much of his current situation has been molded by poor lifestyle choices that were just coping mechanisms. He now finds himself in a serious existential dilemma, where he is very aware that he is not living well, but feels helpless to change it. I predict if he continues on this trajectory, he will suffer an old-age experience like my father's.

    I can tell you emphatically that the kind of aging everyone worries about tends to begin around age 30. Wrinkles start to appear, the skin loses its elasticity and tone, untrained musculature begins to sag and atrophy. The natural physiological predisposition, and eventual inevitability, of having three times more muscle than fat begins. Muscle mass diminishes every year around age 30 and fat mass can increase much more easily. Eyesight and hearing become less sharp and acute. Your bones can become thinner and brittle. Your overall energy, stamina and endurance will decline yearly as well, making it increasingly more difficult to maintain a stressful, busy, and over-scheduled life. Biochemical and hormonal levels that mark our young adulthood start to steadily decline.

    Metabolism also slows as we age. The immune system, the nervous system, the hormonal-regulating system and biochemistry—these systems all diminish in capacity as we age; and this diminishment is well underway by age 50. If you are over 50, then you no doubt are already experiencing this.

Disease and general compromised health tend to increase. The question here is separating the maladies that come with age, from those that are influenced by modern lifestyles, or the ones that are simply the by-product of living longer lives. We underestimate the power of lifestyle in keeping disease at bay as we age (such as heart disease and cancer).

For instance, one of the founders of the prestigious Johns Hopkins Medical School, William Osler, noted that in seven years at John Hopkins, he saw a total of four angina cases. Over a span of ten years at another hospital , he saw *no* cases of angina. Today, cardiologists at hospitals in normal size cities likely see that number every hour! Research shows that, since the turn of the twentieth century around 1900, the incidence of heart attacks has doubled every two decades. Most experts speculate this has happened for three very specific reasons. 1) The pace of life has increased with unhealthy stress levels, 2) our diets have changed substantially, and 3) our activity levels decreased.

Having shared these facts about aging, let me add that I've been around long enough see how adapting a healthy lifestyle can delay the effects and symptoms of aging by decades. Conversely, by not taking conscious control of your life and of healthy lifestyle habits, you inadvertently invite accelerated and premature aging. You likely have good habits you've been practicing for years. You can leverage these for a better quality of life in the second half of your life.

There is plenty you can do besides passively enduring the aging process. And "do" is the key word. Staying youthful requires action and engagement, not just wishful thinking. Transformation and change do not have be negatives. But they do have to be accepted. From age 50 onward, you need to embrace the notion that you have many skills and abilities at your disposal merely from having lived this long. Focus on what is realistic for you.

Embrace that aging does not have to be defined by declining physical function. It can be about unlimited possibilities and new discoveries.

CHAPTER 1.

Fear of Aging

Fear of aging is actually quite common. I am not talking about a fear of those final elder years when the body or the mind has gone and death is near. I mean fear that much of life is still right in front of you, waiting to be lived and embraced and enjoyed, only not as a young person. I get so many people writing me who are pining for lost youth and saying things like, "I wish I was young again" or some such sentiment. These people aren't even as old as I am.

Aging is inevitable. All you can control is your lifestyle going into it, and your perspective about it as well. Many people want to deal with aging by denying it or to attempting to prevent it by any means available. That makes no sense.

I received I one letter recently from a woman asking me about "life extensionists". Here is that letter:

Dear Coach Abel

I hope you can give me some advice. I am a 47 year old female and I am considering a local life extensionist Coach and doctor. They want to prescribe Growth Hormone among other things as part of their package. There is also a laundry list of supplements they want to sell me and I am a bit skeptical of those. I'll do anything to not look my age. I've had cosmetic surgery, botox, liposuction, and I exercise and eat right. But I can see that I am starting to look older and I hate it. I mean, I feel fine more or less, and I know I can't be like I was when I was younger, but can you recommend any supplements or regimens as part of this anti-aging approach? The Life-extensionist package will be about $3,500 per month and that is a lot of money for me. But I also do not want to look like I am 50 in three *years. I'm terrified of that. Any advice or recommendations?*

I tried to persuade this lady to change her perspective on aging. I don't even like the term "anti-aging." It's a marketing term full of innuendo. Imagine using the term "anti-aging" for someone about to enter their teen years, as if to imply you can stop puberty or something. It makes no sense.

You may be able to do things surgically and cosmetically to "look younger." Those only mask that you are in fact "aging." I would rather be real about it and make the point that what you really can do is just not invite accelerated or premature aging. Advertisers focus on youth culture but our population as a whole is actually getting older.

That aside, chronological age is not nearly as important as biological age when it comes to health and well-being. Fighting aging just makes no sense because it puts you at odds with yourself, and that is no way to live in wellness. At some level, fighting aging is about fear of death. Accepting aging should constantly remind you how important it is to embrace life.

There is an old saying I find to be true:

> "You are as young as your faith, as old as your doubts; as young as your self-confidence, as old as your fears; as young as your hopes, as old as your regrets."

I love this saying. Anyone over 45 years old should have this written down somewhere readily visible. Fear produces exactly what you don't want. There's a Zen expression, "What you fear will appear." Nothing invites premature, accelerated aging faster than fearing it. It makes no sense to fear an inevitability of life.

If you filter your perception of aging through fear, you deny yourself many benefits that come with your maturity. Age is a natural transition, whether it be from infancy to childhood, childhood to teen years, teen years to adulthood, and adulthood to living to age 50 and beyond. It does not have to be a time of lost dignity and diminished self-worth. To fear these transitions of age makes no sense and only creates a subconscious foundation of stress and resistance.

CHAPTER 2.

Biological Age, Chronological Age and Psychological Age

Baseball legend Satchell Paige—whose performance in baseball defied time—famously said, "How old would you be if you didn't know how old you were?"

We actually have a way of making an educated guess on this very thing. It's known as biological age. Let me say up front that the concept of biological age is not hard science by any means. It's a social scientist's tool and its formulae vary because of this. Biological age, versus psychological or chronological age, is a very useful tool to consider if you want to inform yourself about how various lifestyle habits impact you. It will tell you a lot about how well you are, or are not, aging.

So let me define a few terms here for you:

Chronological Age

How old the calendar says you are.

Biological Age

How old the your internal cellular processes and absence of disease says you are.

Psychological age

How old you feel, based on things like contentment, absence of stress, absence of illness, world-view, etc.

Even though this formula is more or less a social

scientist's and psychologist's tool, it is still amazing to me how many people my age and older are not even aware of the concept of "biological age."

The biomarkers of aging—things like muscle mass, strength, sex hormone levels, blood pressure, bone density, hearing, immune system vitality, the ability to use and metabolize sugar, body temperature regulation, and even cognitive function—all these things can be improved even later in life. I recently saw on headline news a report on a study that showed that people who read a lot live longer, live better, stay sharper, and suffer less dementia, including Alzheimer's.

The diminished capacities of aging can be slowed. They do not need to just be accepted as inevitable. They are not assumed certainties of the aging process, especially when you are still in your fifties and sixties. The way to improve these biomarkers is with sound healthy lifestyle choices and medical intervention, when and if necessary.

To be sure, aging is indeed a very complex process. You can't just answer a questionnaire to predict when you will die, or how well you will, or won't, age. Obviously individual genetics level plays an important role. However, suffice it to say, that there are plenty of people who wake up to life later in life, sick and tired of being sick-and-tired and want to do something about it. I coach many people who are more energetic, vibrant and robust at age 50 than they were in their late twenties.

When I wrote the original piece about 'The Platinum Club,' we received overwhelmingly positive feedback from people who identify with the notion of aging youthfully and being age-tastic. Conversely, there are others who are still chronologically young, but their inner physiology is that of a person in their sixties or seventies.

I know a lot of former athletes who traded early performance for later pain and body break-down. My own shoulder osteoarthritis, and two damaged discs in my lower back, likely could have been avoided by different lifestyle choices when I was younger. We cannot go back and turn back the clock. We must deal with the facts of "what is" as we age.

The point is that time does not affect all of us the same way, and the realities of biological aging are much different and more complex than simple chronological aging.

Recently I was watching an episode of the show "Ballers" featuring Dwayne (The Rock) Johnson as a retired football player turned agent. His character uses med to manage pain from his past playing days. In this particular episode he gets an X-Ray on his hips as part of his arrangement to keep getting pain meds prescriptions. The doctor comes back and tells him "You need hip replacements...now." He argues, "That's impossible, it's just a little pain and stiffness, I just need some meds." The doctor refuses. Johnson's character replies, "That's impossible doc, I'm only 41." The doctor says back to him, "Maybe the calendar says you are 41, but your hips think you are 85."

It is a fictional scene, but true. I know a lot of former athletes who traded early performance for later pain and body break-down. For me, my shoulder osteoarthritis, and disc issues in my lower back could likely could have been avoided by different lifestyle choices when I was younger.

Physical wear and tear is not limited to contact sports or resistance training. Many marathon runner clients of mine have the leg muscles, cardio fitness and respiratory health of someone half their age, but their knees and hips require joint replacement surgery. They also have compromised kidney health ordinarily found in the elderly. These people are usually still in their forties or early fifties. Regular exercise can be taken too far; while healthy on one side of the equation, it can accelerate aging on another side of it.

Having said all of that, we can't turn back the clock. We must deal with reality as we age.

A former client and training partner of mine has kept in contact with me over the years. He is about nine years older than me. Each time he would write me after I retired to tell me of some new physical issue he was having. As he aged from age 55 to 60, he just kept injuring himself trying to sustain the training and drug regimen he followed when he was younger. First he tore a triceps. About a year later he tore his biceps on the other arm. Then a year after that, he needed shoulder surgery. He's now had both hips replaced, one knee replaced, needs his the other knee replaced and has had elbow surgery. Every time something happens, he reaches out to me. And every time I tell him to get off all the bodybuilding drugs and growth hormone. He follows my advice for a month or two then goes back to his routine. I finally told him that if he keeps this up he won't be able to exercise or work out at all.

I asked him what is more important, the exercise lifestyle, or taking the steroids to artificially support it. Apparently one of his surgeons asked the same question. He is now off all the drugs and he hasn't been injured since. However, his body now has so much wear and tear that he can't do half the training that would have been possible had he just been realistic.

I can't tell you how many times I've witnessed similar scenarios from my own in the hardcore end of bodybuilding background. Former clients tell me their bodies are falling apart, yet they won't give up the training regimens of their younger days. Many won't get off Performance Enhancing Drugs either, which are much harder on the body after age 40. PEDs were why I walked away from professional bodybuilding once I saw what they were doing to my body. Side effects aside, carrying a lot of extra muscle after age 40 is as hard on your body as carrying around the same amount of fat weight. Yet, since so many former clients still relate to "muscle" being part of their identity, they won't surrender the muscle or the training regimens even though their bodies are falling apart.

Biological age is changeable and malleable. The body is a very forgiving machine, but like most machines, it requires regular care and maintenance to function at its best. Regular physical exercise of the right kind can reverse or even arrest a whole host of the typical things that accelerate biological age: high blood pressure, excess body fat, problematic sugar metabolism, and the effects of sarcopenia. (Sarcopenia is marked mostly by the loss of muscle mass, weakened function of metabolism, hormonal function, and biochemical functions.) To the average aging person, the body loses lean tissue and replaces it with adipose tissue (fat) and this process begins relatively imperceptibly in our thirties. By age 65, almost half of the bodyweight of men and women is now metabolically inactive adipose tissue; double the amount it was in your twenties; unless of course you do something about it.

Decisions you make about your basic happiness and fulfillment will also affect how you age. You are likely to age well if you believe a balanced lifestyle of health and wellness leads to happiness and fulfillment, and you see exercise and eating healthy as enjoyable and not just drudgery.

Of all types of age, psychological age is the most flexible and malleable. Like biological age, psychological age is completely individual and personal. And like biological age, psychological age has a lot to do with the choices you make about how you think, what you think about, your worldview, your belief system, and how well you process emotion.

Your body has natural diurnal and circadian

rhythms which cycle roughly once a day. The closer your daily routine and tempo reflects this natural, biological imprint, the healthier you will be and the more likely you will experience physiological "well-being." When you are in concert with natural evolved biological rhythms you are unlikely to have maladaptive bad habits emerge, where you end up treating effects and not causes.

Psychological age is related to mental and emotional fitness. It means keeping your mind young. This requires taking control of your mental health and engaging in constructive, positive, self-directed thought, and mental activities. Reading about a topic of interest, or learning a new skill—maybe through an online course—are just two examples. Surfing other people's social media pages and involving yourself in petty Twitter wars, even as a voyeur, are not. Psychological health requires controlling your environment whenever you can, and filtering what you see and hear when you cannot.

I'll share a common type of letter I receive as an example. Carol is a 48-year-old former figure competitor who was ready to retire from it. Competing over the last five to six years really did a number on her metabolism. She hired me to help her learn to live a more balanced life and separate herself from the physique competition world into which she had immersed herself for so many years.

Dear Coach

Well, of course it is that time of year again and all the ladies at my gym are gearing up to compete and all anyone can talk about is dieting. I try not to listen to it. Then a few of them even say things to me like, "I can't believe you aren't competing anymore. You're going to miss it." Or they'll say, "If you don't compete how else are you going to make yourself stay in shape and not let yourself go?" Coach – I'm so glad you set me straight with all of this. I see how self-consuming it is for all these women. I can't believe that was me for so many years. And yes for a while there I was still following some competitor social media pages that always seem to make me feel bad about myself and that maybe I should compete again. But why?— just to put myself through hell again? My body just can't take it anymore and I need to face that maturely. It took a while, almost like withdrawal; but I finally deleted all these social media competitor pages. And you were right – I couldn't see how all that was filling my mind with such stress and pressure, all because I allowed it to. And now my mind just feels so "free" if that makes sense. I've taken up reading like you suggested and you know what, my workouts feel so much better now. There's no sense of pressure. It's just fun again. And now that I have other things to think about and do, I get what you've been saying about "letting go of things that hold us back." Thank you for all your support. I finally get it now.

I pointed out to Carol that in no way could "all" the ladies in her gym be gearing up to compete, and just as unlikely that they were all talking diet. I told her this was just her selective listening, that she could do something about it, and that her that feelings of pressure and stress should not be attached the things you love.

Be aware of your sources of stress so that you can recognize and deal with them. Even stresses from your past can have major impacts on your physical health. Like computer malware, consciously or unconsciously, these negative past stress events send out harmful messages in the form of biochemical signals to the rest of your body. Over time, a mindset that is constantly anxious, tense, exhausted, stressed, jealous, resentful and disappointed will have a physiological impact, accelerating your biological aging.

Here's a quick check list of things you can do right now to enhance youthfulness and positively impact your biological age:

- Slow down.
- Don't be in a rush all the time.
- Think of projects in terms of process instead of deadlines.
- Never work to exhaustion.
- Take as many breaks during your day as you need to in order to regenerate. Even a five-minute stretch or a walk around your place of business can help.

- Don't put your meal consumption on the clock.
- Slow down and enjoy meal time; don't eat fast.
- Don't eat too much, which is a lot easier to do if you choose healthy whole foods.
- Avoid processed and pre-packaged food.

I just calculated my biological age from one of the online formulas. I'm 34, not bad for a young man who's 55 chronologically! Based on this, I would say that I know a little something about youthfulness and how to keep it. This is due to a healthy lifestyle and life choices I made...I'm eager to share those with you.

CHAPTER 3.

A New Kind of Youthfulness

"The more sand that has escaped from the hourglass of our life, the clearer we should see through it."

- Jean-Paul Sartre

Aging can give us more depth and insights into what matters and what doesn't. It can add clarity and perspective. It can also help us to let go of all the useless things we used to stress about and found so important when we were younger. When framed this way, I'm not even sure "aging" is the most descriptive word. That's why I coined the word "age-tastic."

I define age-tastic as just "the full ripening of youthfulness." I define this new kind of youthfulness as having energy, freshness, and exuberance. It doesn't mean being chronologically young. It doesn't mean "acting" young, or not acting your age. It means having a different *quality* of energy, and appreciating the exuberance that accompanies a love of life, and having the experience to put it all to good use. I think this is what Sartre meant. Aging offers us clarity. Some people are too focused on the "getting old" part to even appreciate this clarity and the gifts that come with it.

There is a marked difference between "youthful" and "young." Youthful applies to mindset. Young people to chronological age only. Keeping a youthful mind leads to having a youthful appearance and youthful physique. Keeping a youthful mind begets this quality of energy, clarity, and exuberance I've referenced. If you keep active mentally and physically, you can stay youthful.

My occupation requires creative energy and constant mental exercise: solving problems for people, writing books, and doing other projects like Podcasts, videos and online courses. These activities keep my mind sharp. Reading continues to provide me the vital information I need to complete these projects. A recent news report said that avid readers tend to live longer, and live better.

Reading helps my mind stays youthful and exuberant. When I read, I take notes, organize them, then often turn those notes into books. Yet I know people as young as me who are on permanent disability for "stress" or for "chronic fatigue" and the highlight of their day is watching TV, reality TV being the worst. This makes the mind lazy and passive, and invites premature and accelerated decline.

Like your physical body, your mental fitness matters to aging well and is maintained with lots of mental exercise. As long as your chosen mental activity is enjoyable (as with my reading, research, and writing), it creates alpha wave patterns in the brain that are calming and soothing. It's a relaxed but prepared state which is believed to be nourishing to the body. In the next chapter, we will discuss the mind-body connection.

Active mental stimulation helps create youthful mental exuberance, whereas mentally passivity can translate into lethargy and apathy. A saying goes, "You don't stop growing because you get old; you get old because you stop growing." Clichés exist for a reason. There is nothing about aging that would prevent you from choosing mentally engaging activities. Memory care centers offer activities designed to engage the mind. My own mother, who is in her 80s and has dementia, goes to a day program based on mental stimulation and engagement.

If you meet aging with joy, imagination and curiosity, then you meet it with vitality as well. The result is that new kind of youthfulness characterized by exuberance and a calm disposition. Your mind-body connection is key to living age-tastically. But you have to first understand what this connection is.

We will consider the mind-body connection in the next section and the additive effects when mental and physical exercise are both practiced as we continue our life's journey.

CHAPTER 4.

Mind-Body and Body-Mind Connection

Most research on aging reflects a common theme among people who age well. They do so by staying active in three major areas: physical exercise, psychological and intellectual challenge (e.g., reading and writing), and having active social relationships. In short, they take care of their bodies *and* their minds. They are "proactive" in the care of themselves, not reactive.

An active mind and active body matter as we age. Age 50 is but the infancy of our aging process toward the final transition of our lives. Creativity and imagination and even wisdom keep you youthful with challenge and purpose, maybe even inspiration. Picasso, George Bernard Shaw, Michelangelo, and Tolstoy lived long lives but productive lives even into their elder years. Michelangelo designed the dome of St. Peter's when he was in his ninth decade of life. Former president Jimmy Carter is in his nineties and still traveling around the US building houses for habitat for humanity. He has had health issues, but conquered them all. I also think of pop-culture television icon Judge Judy, 75 years old and host of the longest running television show in history. Warren Buffet is now 86 and still working. Betty White was still acting in sitcoms in her nineties.

You've likely heard of the mind-body connection. Fewer people consider the body-mind connection. I distinguish body-mind from mind-body to call attention to this: Many will agree that the mind greatly influences the body. I'm among those who say that the body strongly influences the mind. So, when I use either mind-body and body-mind, I do so intentionally. In my opinion, to be age-tastic, you must embrace the notion that your mind influences your physiology, and the converse, your physiology influences your mind. This is a two-way relationship to be sure. Read the following excerpts from real letters I've received. I will reference them again as we discuss mind-body and body-mind.

New Client A

New client "A" writes me and says this:

Dear Coach – I'm so happy to finally be coached by you. I've been thinking about it for a long-time now and I follow you on Facebook and on your Podcasts. And I have a few of your books too. I have in the last couple of years finally started taking better care of myself. My kids are now grown and out of the house and starting their own families. I ran out of excuses and I just started everything slowly on my own. In two years I've lost about 30 lbs and I eat healthier now than I ever have—but as you advise I don't obsess about it either. I work out about 4-5 days per week and I am very involved with my local church. But I want to hire you as my coach. I want to do this better and be better. I like your holistic approach that you consider the mind and the person as well. I like that I can share with you and be accountable to you, but still learn from you as well. I've done well this far on my own and it's not about taking it to the next level or anything hardcore like that. I just know I would feel better with your guidance as I go along. I just feel so great now and I don't ever want to risk something getting in the way of that. What are the next steps to starting one on one coaching with you?

New Client B

New Client "B" writes me and says,

Coach Abel – I am thinking of hiring you as a coach and I want to know if you think you can help me. I'm one of those people you've talked about before. I'm 51 and I'm overweight and I've tried dieting only to gain all my weight back. I try jogging but my knees hurt. I don't like to work out with weights really. I have anxiety and depression and trouble sleeping and so I take sleep meds, both for my sleeping and my anxiety. But the meds make me feel groggy when I wake up so I don't even want to think about exercising. Then when I get depressed I end up eating crap, which only makes me feel worse. Do you think I am someone you can work with?

You can see difference in perception and perspective these two letters juxtapose. If you change your perception and perspective for the positive or negative you change the experience of your body in the process. Perspective shapes your perceptions.

What does all this mean when you start to consider life after age 50? Your self-perception (how you see yourself) is causing physical changes in your body even now. Your perception of your own aging also has similar physiological impact. Appreciation is youthful, regret is aging. Compare the two letters above as clear examples. The mind-body connection is important at any age, but especially so after age 50.

Our body's inner workings are much less

resilient as we begin aging after age 50. Our thinking can exacerbate the physical aging process, or it can help keep us youthful. As the mind goes, so goes the body. There is no doubt that physiology and your mental/emotional worlds are intimately connected; either one can change the other. Being ill can depress you or flatten your mood. Looking forward to each day and what it brings can give you energy and enhance your immune system.

Mind Over Matter

"Age is an issue of mind over matter. If you don't mind, it doesn't matter."

- Mark Twain

We know that just thinking about a past stressful event can release stress hormones in the body. Post Traumatic Stress Disorder (PTSD) manifests itself this way, when a past traumatic event triggers physiologic and emotional reactions. It's amazing to me that in our day and age people don't believe in the mind-body connection. I've had people tell me they don't. But the truth is that the two cannot really ever be separated.

Author Norman Cousins, for whom illness, healing and regeneration was a frequent topic, said, "Belief creates biology." Although Cousins died of heart failure, he lived 10 years longer than expected, and *36 years* after first being diagnosed with heart disease. The quote above appears to be a direct reference to the mind-body connection. Obviously he believed in the connection between the mind and body. So do I.

Aging well requires emotional resilience, embodied by vitality, vibrancy, a youthful spirit, positive attitude, values, and healthy beliefs about aging itself. You accept reality and don't pine away for what once was. Aging well is all about adaptability. Look at those two letters above again. One person "feels" great and wants to expand on that. The other person "feels sick" and her body is the living reflection, hurting and overweight.

Shakespeare wrote this line for Iago in *Othello*, "Our bodies are our gardens, to the which our wills are the gardeners." This applies to aging, either for passive acceptance of it, or for actively participating in it and embracing that phase of your life. You can use physical changes and diminishing physical capacity as a reason to think harshly about your body, or you can marvel at all your body is still able to do for you, and tend to it as an active gardener.

Your beliefs and your thoughts have a lot more power and influence over your physiology than you may realize. The biochemistry of your body can be influenced heavily by your level of awareness and consciousness and the things you think about and how you feel most of the time.

Ghandi put it this way, "Your beliefs become your thoughts, your thoughts become your words, your words become your actions, your actions become your habits, your habits become your values, and your values become your destiny." So your beliefs about this aging process have power to influence you and your body in ways you may never have considered before.

The "Retirement Effect"

In the late nineteenth century, 75 percent of male workers in the US were still working after age 65. Men not working after age 65 were assumed to be disabled. The introduction of retirement in 1935 established a numerical age, 65, as a time at which a person was expected to no longer work. Yet in 1935, life expectancy was 60, which means that most people were working until the day they died.

Retirement established an arbitrary, artificial end to a person's usefulness. "Early death from retirement" is an actual syndrome that has been studied. When someone assumes in retirement that their usefulness is gone they lose their sense of purpose. This is enough to lead to disease, cancers, and even sudden death by heart attack or stroke.

Often a scenario plays out like this: a person who has worked his whole life retires. With few other avid interests, he eats more, drinks more alcohol than before, perhaps using it as a coping mechanism without even realizing it. He gains weight. He becomes slow and lethargic. Within a few years of retirement he has his first heart attack that requires surgery. This often comes with post-op advice to rest and not exercise too hard, making him even more sedentary and likely more depressed. He self-medicates with more alcohol or meds, and within another few years suffers another heart attack, maybe a fatal one.

A satisfying occupation not only keeps you active in productive ways, it can help keep stress level low. Job satisfaction is one of the most key elements that relate to health and reduced risk of heart attack from stress.

The Outlook on Working Out

It's important to stay active and keep a youthful mind. You do that by staying engaged mentally, and by exercising regularly. Being able to work out alone can contribute to a positive mental outlook. Compare the statements, "I have to work out," with "I get to workout." Personally, every day I find myself noting how grateful I am to still be working out at a high level and enjoying my walks in this naturally beautiful area where I live.

My workouts support the mental appreciation I have for them, and the mental appreciation I have for them reinforces my desire in me to keep working out. I haven't even discussed the benefits of endorphins (feel-good hormones) that exercise produces, which further enhances a positive state of mind. The habit of this fitness lifestyle becomes a value, and that value contributes to the "new kind of youthfulness," discussed previously.

How you *think* about physical activity can make the difference between remaining youthful, or feeling and acting "old," as if your best years are behind you. You will notice diminished physical capacities as you age, but your body still has plenty to offer you, and it has wisdom to teach you if you listen to it.

If you view your body as separate from yourself and as a project, then you must change your perception to one where your body is related to your mind and not as only as functional and cosmetic. It takes a desire to start living from an inside-out awareness to be able to tap into the wisdom of the body and rely on it.

As I was writing this section on the connection between mind and body, I ran across a study published in the journal *Gerontology* correlating cognitive health, aging, and leg strength. The authors found that leg strength was strongly correlated to cognitive health. The study subjects with the strongest legs kept their mental capabilities longer. The study ruled out genetic differences by using twins, who have identical genes and similar lifestyles during their formative years. Dr Claire Steves, one of the study's authors, said this:

It's compelling to see such differences in cognition and brain structure in identical twins, who had different leg power ten years before.

It suggests that simple lifestyle changes to boost our physical activity may help to keep us both mentally and physically healthy. [01]

According to the research, leg strength was *the best* predictor of healthy cognitive aging.[02]

Once again we see the heavy influence of the body-mind connection. The study supports that weight/resistance training is an excellent way to keep your mind youthful.

Mental Foundation for a More Youthful Body

Your body can be a barometer for *how* you are thinking, how you are feeling, and how you may be responding to a given situation or circumstance. When the body is in good balance, your mind sends signals of well-being. When the body is out of balance, it sends signals of dis-ease and discomfort. Your body seldom lies, but your ego's interpretations of your body's messages will, if your belief system doesn't filter those interpretations.

What if you manifest a belief, as I have, that these years from 50 onward are the most gratifying years of your life? I recall all the useless things that caused me stress in my younger years. Now I smile at how much of that baggage I have left behind due to my belief in what life after 50 can be. That belief energizes me.

Mood is also important. Mood differs from beliefs but also affects physiology, and vice versa. Have you ever watched a comedy while being really sick, been able to laugh hysterically, and felt a little better right away? Similarly, being depressed or anxious over some life situation can start a cascade of physiologic events that cause insomnia, which itself negatively affects your overall well-being. The stressful event doesn't need to be current for this to occur. It has been shown in research time and time again that merely remembering then focusing on some stressful time in your life triggers unfavorable physiological responses.

How effectively a person manages their moods is a sign of *emotional intelligence*, as studied by Daniel Goleman. This can involve deep understanding of oneself, such that a person can objectively monitor what they feel or think at the moment, and can adjust, based on beliefs. For the purposes of this project, I'll refer to it as Emotional Fitness.

Emotional Fitness is marked by a certain emotional flexibility and adaptability to changing conditions; just as mental flexibility and adaptability are also predictors of aging more slowly. Goleman writes in his landmark text *Emotional Intelligence*, "...the design of the brain means that we very often have little or no control over when we are swept by emotion, nor over *what* emotion it will be. But we can have some say in *how long* an emotion will last."

The emotionally fit possess a capacity for enjoyment and for regular laughter, having a certain degree of self-sufficiency, and an ability to solve your own personal problems. But it also means processing emotions well and not trying to repress, suppress, ignore, or medicate them away.

People with sound Emotional Fitness will teach their bodies to age well and to be age-tastic, by nourishing their bodies with healthy thoughts and positive emotional sentiments; mindful nutrition if you will. That is hard to do if you are always reacting to being over-burdened, and over-stressed. People whose mindsets are founded mostly upon negative emotions and imprints, like anxiety, anger, hostility, frustration, depression, insecurity etc – these people instruct their bodies to age poorly; because they mentally nourish their bodies poorly (Youthful mind = positive mind. Old mind = negative mind). Mental fitness goes a long way to aging well.

Studies show that *intelligence* correlates with aging well too, which makes sense if you consider intelligence will likely lead to making wiser lifestyle choices throughout life.[03] But let's consider *wisdom*—being prudent, knowing yourself and how the world works—to be even one step beyond intelligence in preventing premature and accelerated aging. This makes it easier to know your stress triggers and respond to them more preemptively and preventively.

Taking care of your mind's health and well-being is as important taking care of your body. After age 50, mental and emotional fitness matters. There is a reason the expression "worried to death" exists. On the other hand, when you have a positive harmonious connection between your inner and outer worlds, you will feel joy, contentment and to a large extent you will feel youthful.

Too many people pay lip service to the mind-body body-mind connection but then live a life ignoring it, or understanding very little about what it really means in practice. After age 50, a healthy *mind affects the body* in healthy ways and a healthy *body affects the mind* in healthy ways. To be making the best of both your body and your mind, by keeping both active and engaged, you age well and go a long way toward being age-tastic.

Negative Body and Mind Dynamics that Affect Aging

- Depression, chronic worry, anxiety, chronic low or negative emotional predispositions
- Inability or unwillingness to process and express emotion, unwanted or negative emotions especially
- Heavily judgmental of self and others
- Job dissatisfaction
- Feeling helpless

- Fear of change
- Mental rigidity
- Loneliness
- Lack of social connections and social network
- Lack of regular *daily* routine
- Lack of regular *work* routine
- Inconsistent exercise
- Lack of exercise
- Overworked, over-scheduled, busy-ness (what I call "tail-chasing")
- Financial stress, debt
- Negative imprints from the past: Regrets, guilt
- Negative emotional foundations: Irritability, frustration, anger, hostility
- Disrupted sleep or insomnia

Positive Mind-Body Body-Mind Dynamics that Keep You Youthful

- Personal sense of well-being, contentment, joy as a state of being, not merely as a state of mind
- Job satisfaction: sense of purpose
- Sociability: Ability to establish new relationships and keep them
- Laughter: Ability to laugh freely and easily, to find humor in things
- Satisfactory sex life
- Satisfying long-term spousal type of relationship, whether romantic or platonic (non-sexual)
- Optimism, especially about your life and how you feel about your future
- Ability to express feelings freely and ability to process all emotions
- Living within your means, and having a sense of financial stability

- Satisfying hobbies or vocations
- Ability to enjoy leisure time/free time
- Good sleep hygiene
- Taking regular vacations
- Feeling in control of your life
- Regular *daily* routine
- Regular *work* routine
- Regular exercise
- Whole food diet strategy (most of the time)

Stress

North Americans stress about pretty much everything, and then try to control everything. This is not a path to wellness. After 50, our bodies are not as physiologically resilient in handling stress. So the key is reducing external stressors that create a stress response in the first place. No one can function well, do well, be well or age well or be age-tastic when the body is in a continual cycle of stress response of constantly secreting adrenaline and cortisol.

These hormones are the major catabolic hormones that break down tissues. Extended and prolonged secretion of them leads to disease and to premature, accelerated aging. Our bodies' physiologies evolved to be able to handle acute levels of stress but not to handle chronic levels of it. This is our modern dilemma: all the abundance and convenience of life man has never known before, combined with higher stress levels than man has never before known.

The connection between aging and stress hormones is well-established in the research; and this includes premature and accelerated aging as well. Emotional stress and anxiety can lead to premature or accelerated aging. Experiments with animals clearly show that putting test animals under stress results in them aging more rapidly. Anxiety is the enemy of creative assertive energy. Anxiety and worry are obstacles to self-improvement. In short, stress itself doesn't lead to premature aging and illness, but surrendering inner flexibility and adaptability to stress does.

To me, the accrued consequences of ongoing stress are that these consequences look very much like getting old quicker. Think about it: high blood pressure, ulcers, impotence, depression, illness and diabetes are all common attributes of the elderly. Whenever the body feels stress whether real imagined, the release of stress hormones triggers biochemical reactions identical to those associated with the aging process.

So it stands to reason, that to engage a healthier hormonal and biochemical profile as we age, we need to reduce the types and amounts of hormones that accelerate that process. Therefore stress-reduction in general is one way to stay youthful. Surrender a need to control everything, and 'don't sweat the small stuff.'

In fact, in most stress-management courses, letting go of a need to control everything is *the* single most important principle for reducing stress. Trying to control every little detail of your day and your life will lead to stress. For example, you could be an effective time manager and have a disciplined and structured routine (which I recommend) without being inflexible and rigid. You must learn to be able to go with the flow to a certain extent, and to realize that some details are not worth the energy required to control them. We call this level of affect "emotional resilience" and it is a sign of mature emotional fitness that is so important to staying youthful.

Too much stress isn't always the problem. Sometimes a lack of healthy physiological or psychological coping with the stress is. The individual way you personally filter what is going on in your life determines how stressful you find a situation.

Maladaptive coping strategies like overeating, binging, alcohol abuse, and mood altering drugs are all "choices" that tend to contribute stress long-term, even though they seem to offer immediate or short-term relief. These coping behaviors are merely an attempt at making symptoms go away, not a way to deal with causes. Learning to reduce or eliminate causes of stress, or at least, reducing the intensity, is far better than medicating them.

Sleep is a natural stress reducer. You will see sleep referenced throughout this project (and other works of mine) for its positive effects on overall health.

Research also clearly shows that contact with nature, and natural surroundings, and so on, almost always reduces stress. Something as simple as trail walks, or something more involved, like bird-watching for instance, can remove and reduce stress, and therefore be a natural means to combat accelerated and premature aging.

Simple Habits

As far back as 1965 research by Lester Breslow and Nadia Belloc showed that secrets to longevity, health, and well-being boiled down to some very simple and obvious lifestyle habits.[4] The habits they listed were:

- Sleeping seven to eight hours per night

- Nutrition: Eating breakfast every day, and not eating between meals.
- Maintaining fairly stable (not fluctuating) bodyweight
- Regular physical activity, including things as minor as gardening
- Not smoking
- Moderate drinking only

When analyzing their statistics, Breslow and Belloc noted that a 45-year-old man (in 1965) who observed up to three of these habits could expect to live another 21.6 years. But, someone who followed six or seven of these habits could expect to live 33 more years. In other words, just eating breakfast, regardless of its composition, and just getting a regular good night's sleep could add 11 years to someone's life. They also found that a person of middle age—considered by them to be someone between 55 to 64—who practiced all seven of these good habits to be as healthy as adults as young as 25 to 34 who, by comparison, only followed one or two of these healthy anti-aging lifestyle habits.

This comparison held across all age groups studied. Someone at age 75 who practiced all of these 7 aging-preventative habits was comparable to someone in their 30s or 40s who neglected these habits.

Their conclusions have been replicated over and over again since this 1965 study. It's not magic or the sexy stuff that will sell to consumers or make for breaking headline news. It's just mundane, common sense stuff that leads to healthy balance and wellness. My interest in these data is not merely the quantity of years added, but the quality of those years.

The research is pretty clear that age doesn't have to just happen *to* you. To a large extent, how well or poorly you age depends on the genetic cards you've been dealt, although not absolutely. You can make conscious, deliberate, purposeful lifestyle choices that will not only add years to your life, but will also add life to your years. The overall message from the Breslow-Belloc research was that people with solid lifestyle habits (although perhaps boring habits to some) could not only expect to live 30 years longer, but healthier as compared with those who without good lifestyle habits. It is clear that a lifestyle of balance, consistency and regularity of diet, exercise, and sleep, is likely the most important step to delaying the ravages of the aging process. Research continues to support and reinforce its major conclusions five decades after this ground-breaking study,

Notice the recurrence of sleep as a contributor to good health. It continues to come up in the research in how to control weight, stay youthful and healthy, and maintain vitality. It also reboots the system and is completely restorative mentally and physiologically. But sleep is also more easily disrupted as we get older. Therefore, having healthy sleep hygiene habits in place goes a long way toward preventing accelerated or premature aging.

Research has shown that people over age 65 who take lots of vitamin supplements and who are rigid about eating strictly health foods only did not gain any advantage at all in terms of life expectancy beyond others who applied good lifestyle habits. The message here is obvious: just keep it simple; know that lifestyle habits are more important to aging well and to preventing accelerate and premature aging; than are any magic supplement solutions.

Sedentary lifestyle and smoking, especially a combination of the two, are the easiest predictors of early death. In fact research is now suggesting that a sedentary lifestyle is akin to smoking one or two packs of cigarettes per day.

In conclusion...

There are advantages that aging offers that you will never see if you perceive aging as some kind of curse, or if you glorify your youth for more than it actually was. The key to keeping a youthful mind is engaging in life, not withdrawing from it. Through wiser lifestyle choices, deliberately engaging your mind and your body in positive ways, and by exercising both body and mind, you can positively influence your overall health. Your body and metabolism can be nurtured by constructive, productive thoughts, feelings and behaviors.

CHAPTER 5.

The Importance of Awareness

Perception, Perspective and Other Important Concepts

In this section we are going to discuss some of the more metaphysical and esoteric elements of personality. Some people would call these concepts "spiritual." I'm not so sure we need to define these concepts under any specific unifying theme, but they should be included in the larger discussion on aging.

Studying, then practicing, these concepts changed my life for the better. I begin this discussion knowing that many of you will read this section with skepticism, or disbelief. I encourage you to just read and consider the arguments nonetheless.

How does spirituality factor into the aging process? Spirituality—not necessarily religion—cannot be separated from your physiology. Many of the letters I receive are from people in their mid-to-late forties or early fifties, who are going through some kind of existential dilemma. Around this point in life, many people seek deeper meaning.

As you consider the aging proposition, think about this famous cliché: "It is important at this time to remind yourself that you are not a human being having a spiritual experience. You are in fact, a spiritual being having a human experience." This self-organizing premise does not have to be religious in nature, although it certainly could be.

You may choose to call spirituality "personal growth" or "deeper self-awareness." Whatever you call it, this deeper self-connection is intimately connected with your physiology. Expanding on the previous section, where we discussed mind-body, this would be mind-body-soul. Deeper connection and communication from within yourself goes a long way toward restoring or keeping balance, which then leads to an *experience* of wellness, and quite possibly wellness itself.

So often, medicine is prescribed as a convenient solutions for problems—like anxiety—whose root cause is not medical. Often the ultimate solutions to personal angst are not best treated with medicine. Sometimes, the best solutions are more about conscious and deliberate personal change, or as I have said before, solutions are often about 'going deeper so you can live better.'

I receive letters from clients and non-clients in their late forties or early fifties and who just are not happy with their station in life. To me, only some real soul-searching and a shift in thinking to deeper awareness are going to help people truly move beyond the helpless feeling of being "stuck."

Here is a sample letter from "Linda":

Dear Coach Abel,

I have followed you for some time on Facebook and I have a few of your books. I'm not sure if you can help me and I'm not even sure why exactly I'm writing to be honest. I mean, it's not that I couldn't stand to lose a few pounds but I'm not all that interested in making it my life either. But I do think I could use some help just to get me back up on my feet and into having a life again. It just feels like you may be someone who could help me with that in a coaching relationship if you do that sort of thing? About 5-6 years ago my husband of 34 years sprung it on me that he had been having an affair for a couple of years and that he was leaving me. We have three kids and 4 grandkids. Our family has been torn apart by it all. But it's really taken a toll on me. And now it's almost 6 years later and it still feels like it just happened. Sometimes I don't sleep for days when I get thinking about it all. I have sleep meds, strong ones really but they make me feel like crap, just less crappy than it feels when not sleeping for a week or more. I've tried online dating to get back out there again but that only added to the nightmare; as I had five really bad experiences and decided that is just not for me. And it's not like I want to be alone forever either, but I just feel stuck right now. I do like my job and my apartment so those are some positives.

But I just want to be able to let this go and move on. I'm thinking that maybe a fitness regimen and really some ongoing coaching could help me do that. And I do know that it's all something I have to do for myself. I don't expect you to have magic solutions. I just need help and I know it. Is this something you could do – I mean could we do the coaching to help me this way? Thank you for your time.

Letters like Linda's are not rare for a fitness Coach to receive. One of the reasons I am writing this book is because of the numbers of letters I get from both men and women in our 50-and-over age group who are simply struggling with where they are at in their lives. And while fitness can certainly be a part of a better life, often it goes deeper than that.

Awareness

"When it comes to staying young, a mind-lift beats a face-lift any day."

- Marty Bucella

Awareness, in my usage, is very similar to mindfulness, which has been defined as "bringing one's complete attention to the present experience on a moment-to-moment basis."[05]

Being present in the moment is a certain state of natural intelligence. To lose being present right now, to lose your awareness of your situation and yourself is to lose that natural intelligence that most wild mammals rely on for survival. Perhaps more to the point of this book, maintaining (or transforming) your body as you age first requires your awareness. Especially after age 50, you shouldn't make a physical transformation be first about your appearance, your weight or your diet. Make it be first about your awareness and being present so you can make consistent healthy choices moving forward.

Our modern world is more concerned than ever with appearances and "staying young" than how we feel inside. In a culture that glorifies youth and pays little attention to age—or even makes fun of it—it's more difficult to embrace aging as a positive, transformative experience. Botox and cosmetic surgery might make you look younger, but won't help you embrace reality. Self-regard, autonomy, productivity and contribution are attributes that last.

You can easily adopt a perspective that your fifties are the youth of your later years. How you view this decade will have tremendous impact on how you experience your progressing years. We could categorize this consciousness as 'aging with awareness' or 'intelligent aging,' to give it a conceptual label.

As you age, you will likely find that you have to discard former interpretations of the world and of your life; and invite new and different realities to replace these past, prior world views and mental constructs. In my own past, I forged my career in competitive bodybuilding, where my physique was my billboard and business card. This served me well for a very limited number of years. Had I stuck with body image as a priority, I am sure I would have created a lot of useless stress for myself, and would not have been able to branch off into so many varying directions and help as many people as I have.

I have witnessed close friends and casual acquaintances die young because they could not surrender their body image as a priority. They abused steroids, and other industry-associated pharmaceuticals, to support their warped self image. While steroid abuse may have minimal negative effects at younger ages, it becomes an internal assault on the body of someone abusing them beyond their mid-forties.

In my experience, the most powerful influences on how you will age come from your level of awareness, or lack of it. Because aging happens so slowly, it takes place outside many people's field of awareness, until it is too late to do much about it. I receive letters from people who tell how they started gaining a little weight during their early forties and didn't think much about it then. Now, in their later forties or early fifties, that "little weight gain" has become a substantial 40, 50, even 60 lbs. or more. Many of them will say things like, "I don't know how I even let this happen. It is like I woke up one day and realized 'I'm really fat and overweight.'"

You cannot control whatever happens outside of your field of awareness. Our bodies are always communicating with us, and our thoughts and feelings are sending constant messages to our bodies as well. Being aware opens the flow of that communication from body to mind and mind to body.

Better, deeper awareness not only has the power to change how you experience aging, it can influence the aging process itself. You act the way you think. When you are consciously aware, thinking positive and constructive thoughts, usually positive self-enhancing productive behaviors follow. When overarching mental patterns are destructive and negative, destructive actions and behaviors inevitably follow.

How you see yourself has a decisively impactful influence on how your body functions, and on your health and well-being. And well-being is always connected to well-doing, and well-thinking.

At any age your quality and abundance of life depend on your sense of personal identity. Think of yourself as old and aging, and that will likely be your experience. If your sense of identity is primarily tied to the appearance of your physical body, then your quality of life will likely diminish as you age. Think of yourself as free and liberated from the vanities of youth, benefitting from your wisdom of experience, and you will likely live youthfully and age gracefully.

After age 50, we have the benefit of a lot of life experience that *should* bring wisdom with it. But if you aren't open to it, you won't find it.

My life experience is the major contributor to my happiness. I am no longer concerned with the vanities of youth. I know who I am, what I'm about, and this constantly informs me in very constructive ways. I no longer allow my ego to distract me from my interests or things I want to accomplish. My age has led me to a different level of depth that I relish. I find this youth of my elder years to be very liberating and invigorating. I am able to let go of *what was* for the fascination with *what is*.

Knowing that I will get older, and knowing all the potential risks of that that are outside my control, just makes me appreciate each day even more. I am thankful that I am "aware" of this and can invest myself in every single day. In fact as part of my morning prayers, I say a prayer of gratitude that I'm aware that I'm conscious of this. You could say that my practice of awareness has me almost always practicing being "present" in the moment, for the moment.

Awareness is always marked by a mind that can continually be present and adaptable. Awareness is the opposite of meeting each situation or circumstance with pre-conceived notions and rigid viewpoints. Awareness cannot be practiced if you are always in reaction mode. If you objectively self-assess, you may find that you are not very adaptable mentally right now.

Objective self-assessment is the first step to awareness. The second step is paying more attention to your thoughts. The third is to challenge thoughts that don't serve you well. Fourth, consciously replace these thoughts with a more constructive, self-nourishing frame of mind. We call this "self-directed thought." With awareness training, you simply make your mind more proactive than reactive.

So in terms of better awareness, the key to having a productive aging experience is in being flexible in thoughts and feelings. Now that I am in my mid-fifties, I have often witnessed proof of the importance of flexibility in thought. The most rigid thinkers seem to be having the hardest times and life experiences, especially in matters of health and well-being. I meet so many people my age who are enjoying the happiest times of their lives *right now*. Maximizing your current situation has a lot to do with this.

Philosopher, scientist and renaissance man Sir Francis Bacon had this to say about mental rigidity and its influences on aging, way back in the 1600s:

the crotchety old people are those "who object too much, consult too long, adventure too little, and repent too soon."

The youthful mind is marked by adaptability. Adaptability here means freedom from conditioned responses, especially responses that no longer serve you. An example would be automatically thinking that a better body means a better life for you. Another example would be in thinking that you can't do anything about your current circumstances.

Self-talk also matters. There is a huge difference between saying in your own head "I'm too tired to do that" (temporary) versus "I'm too old to do that." When you begin self-talk statements with "I am," you need to be careful how you complete those sentences. Your thoughts are powerful things. Guard them. The word "old" carries mental connotations that can change how you feel in the moment and long term. Concentrate on "I am" statements about youthfulness.

Your mind will believe and follow "I am" statements made in your mind. The mind doesn't compromise on "I am" statements. So when it comes to your internal "I am" statements, it's important to make statements that describe your momentary situation, not define you as a person. "I'm too tired to do that right now" is a transient state that will change. "I'm too old to do that" is a self-defining statement not really subject to change. These mark the differences between flexible and rigid thinking.

Take a look at these two letters below and compare them. Both letters come from people in their early fifties. One letter shows flexible youthful mind and the other reflects the mental rigidity that invites premature, accelerated aging.

Letter A

Hey Coach:

I just wanted to write you and thank you for all you do. I've read a few of your books and always like them. A few months ago I read your HardGainer's Solution, and since then I've been following the workouts in that book. I'm 58 and I have a few physical restrictions to training—who doesn't at our age, right? I've been working out my whole life and I was looking for something sustainable for me to suit my age and where I am at. I am loving the HGS workouts and I am actually seeing progress as well and without pain. I've also been reading a lot of the books you have mentioned in your Podcasts, like "Drive" and "Talent is Over-Rated" and your own book "Your Truth is Calling." If you have any other books you can recommend to keep my mind sharp, please let me know. I just wanted to touch base and say how happy I am with HGS and to tell you we're never too old to keep learning. Keep up the good work. I look forward to reading your book "Physique After 50" next.

I include this letter, not because the writer endorses my books, but because it illustrates the mental flexibility and adaptability I've been discussing. The letter talks about a search for a sustainable training program, and talks about reading some books just because I mentioned them. Between the lines you can determine that his mind is open and his overall tone is positive. Now contrast this letter to the next, below.

Letter B

Dear Coach Abel

A friend of mine suggested I write to you. He has tried your products and he swears if anyone could help me you could. A little bit about me is that I am 54 years old, I don't get much exercise because my joints always hurt. I am really overweight because I have Type 2 diabetes. I take metformin for that and I also take medication for my high blood pressure as well. I smoke a bit but not too much to have it be causing me any health issues. I try to stay away from carbs especially fruit and things like that because of my diabetes. My doctor says I really, really need to lose weight, at least 50 lbs or so, but I really don't know how to go about it. Even walking hurts my knees. Any ideas?

We see some rigid, inflexible thinking in Letter B. This person writes about his problems with excuses built in. I wrote back saying the excess weight isn't because of the Type 2 diabetes. The Type 2 diabetes is a result of the excess weight. I also corrected the statement about avoiding fruit, that by eating healthy whole foods such as fruits, potatoes, rice, oatmeal, and vegetables, he could perhaps reduce the medications and some of the inflammation causing joint pain. Lastly, I replied that smoking any amount is unhealthy.

It would seem mine were all logical arguments. I was surprised to receive a reply attempting to refute all the advice I'd provided. The excuses included that there was not enough smoking to contribute to health issues, and that it actually helped relaxation. The reply went on to question my advice to eat carbs regularly, and expressed insult that I suggested that the Type 2 diabetes was due to overweight and not the other way around.

Letter B is an example of rigid inflexible thinking. This plea for help is disguised as a search for affirmation of current beliefs. There's not sufficient flexibility of thought to even consider different ideas and approaches. Compare to the first letter. You can read that its tone is more about helplessness than it is about an open-minded search for solutions. The person writing Letter B doesn't realize that change isn't possible until the victim mentality is abandoned.

CHAPTER 6.

Insight, Intuition, Introspection, and the Benefits of Solitude

After decades of living experience (if we are lucky), we learn our internal cues are the ones we should be directing us. We call this "insight" or "intuition."

Insight provides you with a specific kind of freedom and intelligence that you can't get from reading self-help books or by getting advice from friends. Intuition is self-connecting on a level few people ever experience in their lifetime. Practicing insight and intuition is about trusting yourself as being your own best friend.

Introspection literally means "looking inside." It is honest self-assessment, and lays the foundation for insight and intuition. After age 50, the door is wider ajar than ever to engage some healthy introspection. With practiced introspection, you eventually find that no matter what is going on "around you," you have shelter "within you." It's a place that is comforting, self-regarding, self-knowing and invigorating.

The way to begin practicing insight and intuition is by journaling. Journaling doesn't require deep long essays of the soul. Keep a diary to begin with, and at the end of each day answer the question, "What would I like to say to myself about the day that just ended?" Write out the answer. By doing so, you are being introspective, and beginning the practice of insight and developing your intuition. Once you write down your answer, read it back to yourself. If you this for just a week or two, you will find yourself expanding the conversation. You will find that you are asking yourself even more questions. Write down those questions and answer them as well. Eventually this leads to self-directed thought which are direct reflections of insight and intuition.

You will need enough quiet time so that you can adequately pay attention to journaling and "listen" to your own internal conversation.

Intention and Attention

Think of intention and attention as a beam of light. Intention is about where you point the beam. Attention is like focusing the beam. Intention and attention mutually reinforce each other.

The quality of your life after age 50 will depend on the quality of your attention. You will need both the intent, and the attention to the lifestyle prerequisites to renew and assert your intention to live an active healthy lifestyle. You can dramatically improve your coordination, your strength, your stamina, your vitality, and your mental acuity by making an intentional decision to do so, then following through with the actions and behaviors required to improve them.

Intentionally choosing to embrace yourself, respecting your life and your body, holding it in high regard, at any age will enhance your health and well-being.

Paying attention to your body (not body *image*) will enhance your physiological awareness, putting you more in-tune with physiological changes. You'll be less likely to take it for granted, and more likely to be *intentional* in your habits, such as exercising, choosing to eat healthy, and practicing good sleep hygiene.

The same holds true for your mind. If your intention becomes more about creating and maintaining a youthful mind, your attention will shift toward ways to accomplish that.

You must consciously choose how you age. It is about no longer accepting the default for your mind or body and then living in incessant reaction mode. It requires effort, and more if you're not pursuing it already. Begin by reminding yourself that attention is like focusing a beam of light, and intention is about where you focus that beam. The secret here is about focusing on what you want, not on what you don't. You can't stop the aging process, so resisting the chronological process and what that brings it is futile and a waste of energy. Focus on living better while dealing with the realities of your chronological age. This is what focused attention and intention are all about.

Awareness, with conscious attention and intention intact, creates a mind-body body-mind connection that is directly related to aging well. The more naturally you live this sort of self-directed, inside-out existence, the greater your holistic awareness.

Solitude and Silence

"I live in that solitude which is painful in youth, but delicious in the years of maturity."

- Albert Einstein

"God is the friend of silence."

- Mother Teresa

It can be difficult at any age to carve out time for yourself, to be *by yourself*. Often in our fifties and sixties, we have others to take care of, such as elderly parents and maybe an extended family of grandkids. We have our jobs and other responsibilities that involve being around others. Our modern world is busy, with constant stimulus. This taxes the body at any age, but after age 50 this kind of constant pace can take a health toll. Far too many people underestimate the value of quiet time and solitude to recharge their systems. The ability to be by yourself for some healthy solitude, and the desire for alone time, is a reflection of advanced self-awareness, and a means to stay youthful in mind, body, and spirit.

Silence is the garrison of your sanity and your inner-connected spring of wellness and peace of mind. Trust in silence and solitude. They are the great teachers. I find this is especially relevant at my stage in life.

All you have to do is pay attention to the silence and be okay with the solitude. Leroy Brownlow said, "There are times when silence has the loudest voice." I find that sentence profoundly wise. Practicing silence is simple and doesn't take long. Franz Kafka put it this way,

You do not need to do anything; you do not need to leave your room. Remain sitting at your table and listen. You do not even need to listen; just wait. You do not even need to wait; just become still, quiet and solitary and the world will freely offer itself to you to be unmasked. It has no choice. It will roll in ecstasy at your feet.

People sometimes associate silence and solitude

with 'meditation.' So be it. However, meditation doesn't have to mean sitting in a quiet room with your legs folded in front and chanting. There are various forms of "active" meditation, like long walks, adult coloring book therapy, even a bubble bath with candles. These things tend to clear and rest the mind, keeping it engaged in a calm, peaceful way.

These examples may not fit the classic definition of meditation, but they can serve the same function. The point is that a calm silence serves you well at any age. As we age we accumulate more and more "junk volume" in our minds. There is a ton of accumulated "stuff" we need to learn to just let go of. Quiet alone time is a great way to do just that without conscious effort. Unplug for a while and be silent. Don't get caught in the trap of being a stimulus addict.

Intentional solitude engenders calm, peaceful energy. In a world where the mind is constantly bombarded with stimulus more than ever, this calm peaceful energy is more essential than ever for refreshing, recharging, rebooting, and easing the burdens on your mind. No exhausted organism functions at optimum capacity. Remind yourself of this from time to time, to prompt yourself make room for quiet time, and carve out a little solitude for yourself.

Quiet time is essential for insight and intuition to be properly practiced. To do that, you need to dedicate time, and solitary time if you're able. Practice it for a while and you will begin to understand the "deliciousness" that Einstein is referring to.

Acceptance versus Resistance:
Forms of Energy

Your acceptance or resistance to circumstance, such as your age, create their own forms of "energy," in that they influence how successfully you will handle a given situation or state.

Acceptance is establishing calm peaceful energy as a state of being, and not just a transient state of mind. There are all kinds of situations you have no control over in this world, physiological aging being one of them. Accept it as part of life and your stress levels will decrease substantially.

Part of being age-tastic is the mere acceptance that you are aging and that this is a natural transition. It is what you do about it, a*nd how you think about it* that matters. What, if anything you do about it will have a lot to do with your perspective of it. How you think about this period in your life will determine what you do about it, and these things will determine how you experience this time.

Acceptance helps you keep it real. Uncertainty and insecurity can cause stress, and as we've discussed, the way you deal with stress is the difference between accelerated, premature aging and general overall wellness. So, the way you deal with overall uncertainties in life is either a reflection of wellness, or inviting premature aging. The two ways of dealing with uncertainty in your world are two opposite energy mindsets: acceptance or resistance. The energy of Acceptance represents open-mindedness while the energy of Resistance represents mental rigidity.

Acceptance simply means you know you cannot control other people or every circumstance. You allow for situations beyond your control to unfold as they will, and respond accordingly. Acceptance allows for greater spontaneity and flexibility in terms of your mental, emotional and behavioral responses. This is healthy.

Resistance, on the other hand, is marked by reacting to circumstances by trying to control or fight them. Resistance creates energy that can build up inside you and lead to an emotional implosion, explosion, or both. Resistance can lead to avoidance behaviors and maladaptive coping strategies. It produces frustration, while acceptance produces calm, patient, rational energy. Mental and emotional resistance manifests itself physiologically, not unlike a danger that triggers the natural fight or flight response.

Let me offer this analogy. A non-thrill seeker who decides to try skydiving (perhaps on a dare), will have a much different experience than someone who *is* a thrill seeker and *loves* skydiving. The non-thrill seeker only reluctantly jumps from the plane, with heart racing, screaming with terror, possibly on the verge of passing out. By contrast, the thrill-seeker is yelling in exhilaration. Both engage in the same activity but experience it in very different ways. As you resist the event, you release the stress hormones adrenaline and noradrenaline (catecholamines), whose effects linger after the event is over.

PTSD works this way as well. The person who loves an event does not experience it the same way as the one who is fearful of it. If you can't transition all mindsets from resistance to acceptance, a very challenging task, then learn to avoid scenarios you that you know trigger your resistance mindset and stress response. This is an exercise in stress-reduction. This can even mean making some very hard decisions, such as who to have in your life.

Fear, doubt and anxiety characterize resistance energy. Fear is a terrible motivator because it creates its own form of stress. To fear aging is to invite that very thing feared. This is an example of the expression, "What you fear appears." In terms of attention and intention, you need to shift your attention toward the positive and constructive things that you do want for yourself—rather than focusing attention and intention toward resisting what you don't want.

My mental energies go toward living a healthy lifestyle, not only as a goal, but as a habit. I devote parts of my day toward mental challenge (like writing this book), and my exercise regimen. I don't spend much of any of my mental attention and intention on worrying that I'll be one day older tomorrow. Even when negative circumstances present themselves, I am able to apply the energy of acceptance, dealing with the circumstances directly while maintaining the importance of my healthy lifestyle.

Once this application of energy becomes foundational, circumstances become just what they are—circumstances—and you deal with them as such. This inside-out approach establishes a higher form of wellness, placing you in the most favorable position possible to deal with the natural effects of aging.

Be proactive. Start directing your thoughts toward mentally nourishing and self-supporting ones. This goes beyond such trite expressions as "positive thinking." I advise many of my clients who struggle with negativity to write down, recite, and then practice Philippians 4:8, which says, "Finally, brothers and sisters, whatever is true, whatever is noble, whatever is right, whatever is pure, whatever is lovely, whatever is admirable—if anything is excellent or praiseworthy—think about such things." As you can see here, even as far back as the first century, there's a Biblical reference to the practice of self-directed, constructive and productive thought. This can only be practiced when your energy is in acceptance mode. It is also a great practice for creating and staying in acceptance mode as well. I shouldn't need to point out, but I will anyway—this Bible passage has nothing to do with "religion" and everything to do with sound life-coaching strategy.

Important Lifestyle Factors

Social scientists' research has shown again and again the type of people who live longer and *healthier* in their later years have a higher degree psychological well-being and psychological health in general. One specific piece of relevant research dates back to 1973, when three separate papers were presented at a Duke University Gerontology Conference. This research was, and is still, considered ground-breaking. The 1973 papers outlined the kind of person who would live long and live well to ages 85 to 100, which at the time was less than 5 percent of the population. Research since then has reinforced the proposition that a contented life leads to longevity. Elements of a contented life include:

1. Taking pleasure in daily activities, even mundane ones
2. Regarding your life as meaningful, even if just meaningful to yourself

3. A satisfaction with goals and accomplishments (fewer regrets, or at least minimal focus on regrets)
4. Holding a positive self-image; being a friend to yourself
5. Being optimistic and feeling that life is a gift and always worth living

An expanded list includes:

- Having an interest in current events
- Suffering few illnesses
- A tendency to be free from anxiety
- Not prone to worry and stress
- Routine optimism as part of your overall disposition
- Possessing a sense of humor

The above list has a lot to do with contentment. This is very healthy. Experiencing joy in the simple pleasures of life also helps, as does having higher levels of adaptability to various circumstances. People age well who live immersed in day-to-day satisfaction with their lives. An old Irish salutation says, "May you live as long as you want; and never want as long as you live." I argue here that these two things are intimately connected in terms of quality of life experience and how better, deeper, and higher awareness influences it all.

You can choose not to just "get old" (intention), but you may have to work at it (attention). And working at it is more constructive when you don't fear aging or try to resist it. Accept it for what it is—a transitional period of all life—and then make a conscious choice to get the most out of these wonderful years.

So I'll finish this section by making this point. It's a mistake to live your life from the vantage point of the past or the future, especially if past or future vantage point is attached to negative, anxious energy. Negative energy just keeps you in resistance mode. Being aware—present, and focusing on the present—allows you to create and recreate your world as needs be, and constructively so. Letting your past, or your worries about the future, cloud the present invites premature aging.

CHAPTER 7.

Food Matters

Let's talk about food and food matters. We will look at this first in broad strokes, and then I will discuss the more specific topics of weight-loss and exercise for the over-50 demographic.

I begin by saying that you aren't going to see a lot of ways to calculate and count calories or discussions of carbs, mathematical formulas for dieting, or weight-loss quick fixes here. Simply put, these things just aren't necessary for weight control, nor are they very realistic food and diet strategies. We will discuss here what is actually relevant.

My research into the larger topic of diet has

made me a bit of a historian on diet advice. It's been interesting to see how much the thought on diet has changed through the years, what's actually worked, and what hasn't changed.

In the Victorian era (mid-1800s, to early 1900s) and the decades that followed, many diet and nutrition books were written by doctors who themselves had lived past age 90. There was of course a market for their "secrets" to longevity, just as there is today when a doctor will lend his or her name to a fad diet. Dr. Atkins stands out as the obvious modern example.

If you look at the preponderance of the diet advice of these long-lived doctors of previous eras, their advice for a living longer (at a time when most people did not live as long as we do now) boiled down to a common sense: a simple uncomplicated diet, and lots of exercise. No potions, no pills, no special mixes or magic concoctions, no forbidden, demonized food groups, no mathematical calculations of calories and macros, and all the rest of the modern nonsense surrounding nutrition and diet. Health and wellness are more about "keeping it simple" than they ever will be about fancy, unnecessary, complicated formulas.

Protein and Plants

It is clear from the research that as we age we should place less emphasis on the amount of protein we consume and we should place less emphasis on animal protein "for growth" as well. (See the sections on longevity and vegetarianism in *Modern Nutrition in Health and Disease*.) Our muscles do break down more easily as we age, so it's reasonable to think that this means we should place more emphasis on protein consumption. That simply isn't true. It's actually weight-training that helps slow down the rate of sarcopenia and muscle loss.

Too much protein, and especially constant intake of red meat, is associated with accelerated, premature aging, as well as increased risk for disease. Most text books are pretty clear that vegetarians tend to live longer and have a better quality of life in their later years (*Modern Nutrition in Health and Disease*). However, this does not mean going to the extreme of becoming vegan, which poses its own risks. As usual, some healthy principles can become unhealthy when taken too far.

That said, there is no doubt that a plant-based diet makes the most sense for health, well-being, leanness, aging well, and for quality of life in our later years. A plant-based diet can improve the quality of your life right now. The more of your diet that comes from plants, the less you will have to worry about counting calories and all the rest.

Plant-based diets reduce the risk of most forms of age-associated medical issues, such as heart problems, and diabetes. Most people in the over 50 age demographic who switch to a plant-based diet, consisting of unprocessed whole foods, report clearer thinking and overall greater sense of health and well-being. After a while, they no longer regularly crave other kinds of unhealthy foods. It was that way for me.

Implementing a healthy diet is actually quite easy. Center it on the staples, and on fruits, vegetables, legumes, raw nuts. Eat some egg whites at least once per day and limit animal flesh to twice daily max, and you are well on your way to better inside-out fitness and health.

I want to emphasize that a plant-based diet doesn't mean going vegan. A plant-based diet means that each meal is composed *mostly* of plants, but not necessarily *entirely* composed of plants. We're not talking only about "rabbit food" here either. The starches—like oats, grains, rice, and potatoes—are important. In fact, to me, potatoes are the most sensible food on the planet.

In terms of research, the research supporting a plant-based diet is virtually indisputable. As T. Colin Campbell pointed out in his books, particularly *The China Study, Whole: Rethinking the Science of Nutrition*, and *The Low-Carb Fraud,* you will see certain countries show very low incidence of colon cancer, breast cancer, heart attack, or arteriosclerosis. Japan, Taiwan, Okinawa, Thailand, El Salvador, and certain areas in the Greek Islands are examples. The countries showing the highest incidences of these modern afflictions are the developed countries of United States, Canada, Australia, and Germany.

Looking at the globe, if you plot the countries around the world for their consumption of milk, red meat, and cheese, the very same distribution occurs. In other words the nations with the lowest consumption of high fat foods and red meat are the nations with the lowest disease rates, while the societies who eat the most red meat and dairy are the nations with the most catastrophic rates of heart attacks, cancers, and hardening of the arteries. These are cross-cultural facts not subjective opinion. (See also the text book *Modern Nutrition in Health and Disease.*)

Because metabolism is more vulnerable and susceptible to these ills as we age, these correlations between diseases and food choice merit all of us paying attention to them. If we follow where the research takes us, a plant-based diet with very little red meat, and limited amounts of dairy and other animal flesh, simply makes better sense for our health as we age.

Cultural Considerations

Culture has played a role in the evolution of diet. Early cultural goals for wealth and affluence helped to create many modern physical ills associated with affluence, because what you ate was often a sign of socioeconomic status. The great Potato famine in Ireland (1845-1852) illustrated how important starch staples were to survival, especially for poorer families. But when Irish Immigrants came to America, their perception was that meat on the table in replacement of potatoes and cabbage was an improvement in their family's wealth, social status, and well-being.

Retrospectively speaking, in modern nutrition we know that potato (a healthy starch carb) and cabbage (a healthy fibrous carb) make for much healthier regular fare than does steak and red meat every day. So the Irish "perception" of red meat being a sign of a better life, actually led them to making less-healthy choices for themselves overall.

In other historical eras, produce like veggies weren't valued at all because "they came from the dirt" and these foods were considered "disgusting" at certain levels of social status. Only poor people would these foods. The reason tomatoes were thrown at live performers in the old days was to show disapproval, as these foods themselves were considered "so disgusting." So, cultural perceptions play a role in what we think is healthy and unhealthy. The modern demonization of healthy carbohydrates is another example of faulty cultural impressions that simply aren't true, and that lead many North Americans to making unwise and unhealthy diet choices.

Adding to the problem of food matters in our modern era, because processed food, fast food, and junk food are the cheapest to make and sell, lower socioeconomic groups tend to eat the most of the least healthful foods. That is why socioeconomic status is so closely related to obesity issues.

When you consider a desire for aging well, and food matters related to doing so, it's important to go out of your way to minimize your consumption of processed food, fast food, and junk food. If you are 50 or over, then it is likely that you will relate to the idea that your grandmother's notion of a healthy diet was likely closer to being right on the money than you could have ever imagined growing up. Michael Pollan quipped, "If it comes from a plant, eat it—if it was made *in* a plant (as in factory), don't eat it." If you are eating healthy, whole, unprocessed foods most of the time, then you won't need to consider counting calories and all the rest of the modern day mathematical solutions to diet issues and weight problems.

The Futility of Counting Calories

Let me give you just one example from dozens and dozens of research examples about the futility of calorie counting. Soren Toubro, associate professor of human nutrition at Royal Veterinary and Agricultural University in Copenhagen showed that counting calories is less effective at keeping weight off than just eating an overall low fat higher carbohydrate diet (just like T. Colin Campbell's research, and so many others). In Toubro's research, formerly overweight people who ate this kind of diet for one year regained less than one pound on average. Similar formerly overweight people, who counted calories, *gained 8 pounds*. After two years, the calorie-counting subjects had regained *23 percent each on average*, while those eating low fat, *higher carbs*, and *not counting calories* regained an average 11 lbs.

Since that publication, The National Weight Control Registry—a research group that studies people who have lost a large amount of weight and kept it off for a long-time—has reached the same conclusion: calorie-counting is useless for long-term weight-loss and weight control. Most recently, (as I write this) a 2016 University of Pittsburgh study showed that calorie-counting diet-tracking apps like Fitbit did not help people lose weight at all, especially in comparison to those who did not use such devices.

A Plant, or Made in a Plant?

It's not just junk food, processed food and fast

food we're talking about here. In considering food matters, faux-foods that are represented as being real food, even represented as being "healthy food" and good for you, like health bars and shakes, will never be as good for you as real whole foods like fruits, vegetables, and healthy starch staples like oatmeal, rice, or potatoes.

Bonnie Liebman, director of Nutrition Centers for Science in the Public Interest (Washington DC), said that liquid nutritional supplements are no substitute for real food. "Most of these supplements contain a mixture of water, oil, sugar, soy, milk protein and added vitamins and minerals. Better choices are fruits, vegetables, whole grains, and even yogurt."

These real foods contain fiber and other substances such as phytochemicals that make naturally occurring vitamins and minerals are absorbed more efficiently in your body and work better. In short, liquid supplements, shakes and meal replacements are just processed food marketed to you as "scientifically engineered" (made 'in a plant,' as Michael Pollan warned). "Scientifically engineered" is a marketing term—not a plus for your health and wellness.

So, especially after age 50, if you really want to care for yourself properly, avoid "convenience" foods marketed to you as healthy. They will never be better for you than real whole foods found in the produce section of your grocery store. Say 'no' to health bars and protein shakes, and say 'yes' to whole unprocessed foods. Look at this another way: You don't see labels on the healthiest of the healthy foods in a grocery store. You don't see lists of ingredients on fresh fruits and vegetables. When a manufacturer has to list ingredients on food, and then advertise to you how healthy that food, it *'should be'* a warning sign to you.

Supplements

Most research on aging from the 1990s onward show that people who live longest eat moderately and maintain a fairly constant weight throughout their life. What you don't see in the research is a reflection that those who live longer and live well longer, don't take any vitamins, minerals, and fiber supplements, nor do they follow any kind of specific diet regimen.

Forget specialty vitamin supplements for the aging body. Things like anti-oxidants are always best coming from real, whole foods. Supplements "ride the research" of what antioxidants' function in the body is, but supplemental versions of the real thing simply don't work. Many of these supplements you swallow are nullified by digestive juices in the mouth and stomach long before they get to the cells they are meant to protect. And supplemental forms of things like antioxidants can't possibly be formulated to include all the phytonutrients that are part of whole foods that make these nutrients bioavailable to our cells.

When it comes to vitamins, minerals, and other micronutrients, you need to know that retention and absorption of these micronutrients matter even more than what their function. There is a biochemical complexity to these elements of physiology that cannot be predicted by putting the components in a capsule or tablet and then swallowing them.

Practical Diet Advice

"Eat food, not a lot, mostly plants"

- Michael Pollan

This is about the best diet strategy advice ever given, and I've referenced it in my books before. It suggests a vegetarian-leaning diet approach. There are several varieties of vegetarianism.

Lacto-ovo vegetarian allows for dairy and limited poultry products, like eggs and egg whites. A pescatarian approach allows fish but avoids all other animal flesh. A "flexitarian" approach takes a broader plant-based approach and just limits animal meats and flesh in a more subjective way. For many people, simply eliminating red meat is a general consideration of "vegetarian," although not entirely accurate.

A healthy diet strategy must have three vital components. It must be:

- Psychologically satisfying
- Sustainable in the long-term
- A diet that serves the body

Especially after age 50, a diet should include healthy whole foods that supply a balanced amount of nutrients throughout the day. And remember humans are omnivores. We are evolved to eat a wide variety of foods; but let's not confuse that with eating anything and everything. Obviously I am implying that we eat a wide variety of healthy whole, unprocessed foods. Diets lacking whole foods with plenty of colors and variations tend to be diets that invite accelerated and premature aging. Here is a quick food matters reference checklist to live well after age 50 and beyond.

Limit red meat to once per week and special occasions.

Choose other lean "white" meats but not more than one time per day.

Egg whites are the number one protein choice, and are not animal flesh, so they can be consumed every day, and more than once per day.

Fish is another good source of protein, but consume no more than two to three times per day.

Limit deli meats and other types of cured meats to special occasions only. These are very processed and not good for you on a regular basis.

Don't let more than five hours go by without eating to maintain a good blood sugar level, except for time asleep at night.

Don't eat within 2-1/2 hours of previous meal intake.

Don't eat in rushed and frenzied environments if you can help it. Eat meals in a quiet and peaceful environment. Do not eat meals while multi-tasking.

Eat fiber early in the day. This is particularly helpful because it prevents drops and spikes in blood sugar and sets the start of the day in a positive direction biochemically. Eating fiber early in the day also aids intestinal motility. This helps keep you feeling satisfied longer. For over 30 years, six days per week, I have started my day with egg whites and oatmeal, oat bran or grits.

Sugar tolerance declines with age. Keep that in mind. If you are over 50, you may have learned this from experience. Sugar, desserts, etc after 50 can be very hard on digestion. Regular sugar "treats" can upset a biochemistry and digestive hormonal balance that is already in decline as we age. This doesn't mean that all sugar intake leads to Type 2 diabetes, but it is important to remember that for overall health and wellness value, it is just a good idea to limit these kinds of treats to special occasions, one day per week, or some other arbitrary rule like this.

Wine and beer have some nutritional and metabolic value, but their benefits are over-stated. Hard liquor is not nutritional at all. You should be limiting your alcohol intake as you age.

Hydration stands out as another important factor worth mentioning. Not drinking enough water is one of the most common untreated conditions of old age. Chronic dehydration is a major cause of accelerated and premature aging, but is so easily prevented. This does not mean you have to measure your fluid intake each day, or be in a constant state of diuresis. But it does mean that you should stay conscious of staying well-hydrated if you want to age well.

Having said the above about alcohol and staying well-hydrated, it is also important to note that you should be eating your calories, not drinking them! Stick to water and diet drinks for hydration needs and stay away from liquid calories of all kinds, including energy drinks.

CHAPTER 8.

Weight Loss and Exercise After 50

For thousands of years, deep thinkers knew the wisdom of respecting and honoring your body. The Bible refers to the body as a temple. Buddha said, "Your body is precious. It is your vehicle for awakening. Treat it with care." Regular invigorating exercise is a key component of treating your body with care and not taking it for granted.

Aging is often more than just the result of the passing of years. It is also so often the body's response to the conditions imposed on as these years pass. "It's not the years, it's the miles." This is what I mean when I use the terms premature and accelerated aging.

The word "entropy" is often associated with the aging process. Entropy describes how matters of nature eventually break down from order to disorder. Over the course of a lifetime, each of our cells simply undergoes more damage than it can repair. Think of something like a vehicle for instance. When the outer chassis starts to rust and decay this process cannot reverse itself. By the same token, an aging body's physiology is not just suddenly going to reverse itself and be young again. However, using our vehicle example, a vehicle is kept in a heated garage, driven carefully and in a temperate climate, and serviced regularly should outlast one kept outside, driven hard and not well-maintained. The same applies to how your body ages. In other words, prevention, healthy maintenance, and conscious care go a long way to preservation and delaying the ravages of time.

A recent US CDC research study showed that almost one-third of adults over age 50 simply don't move enough to aid in their own health (CDC Morbidity and Mortality Weekly). These are sedentary conditions imposed on a body that simply invites accelerated and premature aging. The result of not moving enough is ill-health.

Let's remember that up until the latter 1940s, people didn't really need to exercise because daily life was already vigorous and physical. Around 1900, physical labor accounted for about 80 percent of the total calories expended by an individual. Today, most human labor accounts for about 1 percent of total calories expended. That is a whopping difference between the amount of physical activity then and now. And with science and technology making food tastier and more convenient than ever, we have a modern-era dilemma. It is easier to understand how people gain weight than it is to understand why they don't. We live in an era where we move less and tease our taste buds to eat more. When you also factor in that metabolism slows as we age, then it becomes evident that healthy weight management requires consistent due diligence as we age.

You can't just "hope" to not gain fat and lose muscle as you age. Metabolism not only slows with age; it becomes less resilient as well. A study comparing men in their twenties with men in their sixties and seventies found that when younger subjects were fed an extra 1,000 calories per day, their metabolisms were able to handle these extra calories and burn a lot of it off naturally. The older men, however, burned up fewer of the extra calories and gained weight. The study suggested that working out not only helps burn off extra calories (a bit of a no-brainer), but working out also helps indirectly by keeping metabolism optimized and robust (Susan Roberts PHD, USDA Human Nutrition Research Center on Aging, Tufts University, Boston). See also my book *Cycle Diet*.

It seems that maintaining a fairly steady weight throughout life is more important to aging well than whether someone is overweight or underweight. In fact, gaining and losing weight over and over can increase the risk of mortality. People don't tend to think about metabolism and longevity as being connected, but we see in the research gaining and losing weight, weight fluctuation is harder on the body long-term than we may notice. I first started thinking about this when singer Luther Vandross died before age 55. He had been on many diets, and lost and regained weight several times. Since then, I have seen this yo-yo weight syndrome scenario shorten life spans for others. I won't go so far as to say diets lead to an early death, but years of dieting, losing and regaining weight does seem to increase risk of mortality.

From age 50 beyond, exercise should be about more than burning calories. Every time you exercise or work out, you are teaching your body to be stronger. Because of that, your brain, your lungs, your heart, your immune system, and your biochemistry are positively stimulated by this, and they adapt accordingly.

Conversely, if you just do the bare minimum of exercise to get by every day, choosing not to consciously connect with your body through exercise, you forfeit that crucial mind-body connection discussed in a previous chapter. So instead of teaching your body and your body providing feedback, you invite the passivity and lack of awareness that occurs when you become overly sedentary. All these above systems diminish in function and your awareness dulls as well the more sedentary you become.

Exercise is far more than just burning calories. You are truly limiting your scope if burning calories is the only way you've been perceiving exercise. Tap into your body's desire to move and be active for instance. Try to get into a flow with daily activity rather than wake up and go, go, go. You will have a better chance of finding a healthy balance and nurturing vitality. Modern life may require virtually no physical activity, but our bodies do!

Conscious efforts to assert positive, constructive influence over any bodily system produces an overall holistic effect, if you can see beyond the limitation of that single system. The same is true with diet. It should come as no surprise that misuse of your body by being sedentary is a form of personal negligence that invites premature, accelerated aging.

The same is true with mental health. Research is showing that avid readers tend to suffer less dementia and Alzheimer's than do people who do not. Your body and your mind *need* exercise. And it's not just that you must exercise; you should want to. And if you do it just to burn calories and fat then you are missing the grander points of it all.

The body's health deteriorates from lack of use. Lack of exercise causes muscles to become weak making movement and exercise even more difficult. Weight-gain becomes more likely which makes movement and exercise even more difficult. Joint and bone health diminish and can lead to chronic pain, which, again, makes movement and exercise even more difficult. Depression and apathy can set in, which makes you less desirous of exercise. It becomes a vicious cycle.

Chronic fatigue is often a physical consequence of depression, which again makes movement and exercise more difficult and less desirous. Your cardiovascular system and your arteries become more vulnerable to health issues. Most of these negative health implications are considered a natural part of aging, when in reality they are more likely simply the results of not taking care of yourself. It is true also that regular exercise can be a treatment for depression and lack of exercise cause it.

To explain the connection between exercise and depression, you need to understand that the neural mechanism that controls depression often lies with a class of neurochemicals called catecholamines. Catecholamine levels in people who are depressed are abnormally low. Healthy levels can be restored by taking anti-depressants. The natural way to increase catecholamine levels is through regular and consistent exercise, an effect of exercise that is well-documented. During and after exercise, the brain and muscle systems exchange chemical messages, and many metabolic events are configured differently as a result. Part of this biochemical flow during and after exercise stimulates the production of catecholamines.

This may not work as a treatment for everyone with depression of course, but many do not even try this simple, common sense treatment option, at least as an adjunct to medical therapy. Regular consistent exercise is part of proactive health care that will keep you youthful. Being sedentary invites accelerated and premature aging, period.

Exercise is one of the simplest ways to prevent

accelerated, premature aging. Mental and physical neglect, sometimes referred to as "disuse syndrome," accelerates premature aging and aging in general. No demographic is at higher risk for depression, disease, and early death than are people who are completely sedentary. Research with the elderly has conclusively demonstrated that someone who takes up exercise at any age will obtain the same benefits of increased strength, stamina, muscle mass and vitality as younger subjects. In short, exercise can reverse the negative consequences of a sedentary lifestyle. However this should not be confused with a marketing notion that some kind of special exercise program can reverse aging.

In the early 90s, a now-famous research experiment was conducted by Tufts University. The researchers went into a long-term care facility for the elderly and selected some of the frailest residents there and put them on a resistance training regimen. Rather than being exhausted of their frailty, the residents actually thrived. Within about 8 weeks, muscle wasting was reversed and muscle and strength improved by 300%. The residents also improved in coordination and balance. Perhaps most importantly, they experienced a renewed sense of energy and vitality. What makes this whole study remarkable is that the youngest participant in the group was 87 and the oldest participating resident was 96.

The takeaway message here is that resistance training has value at any age. Consider the example of someone who is elderly and afraid to move their body. Their muscles get weak and waste away. I saw this with my own mother. She rarely went outside when she got older. She got weak and then literally *couldn't* go outside. Now that she is in a facility and taking part in various activities, she wants to move around more, so she does. She has reclaimed some strength and mobility again, at least better than before.

If you exercise regularly because you believe it will do you good, then it will. Belief creates biology. If you believe you are too old, frail or sick to exercise, you will prove yourself right. But if previously untrained 87 to 96-year-olds can gain strength and mobility from weight training, then imagine what it can do for you if you begin in your fifties. It is never, ever too late to treat your body well.

Although the Tufts University research clearly illustrated that some of the major symptoms of biological aging can be combatted and improved with consistent exercise, it does not to argue that aging itself can be reversed. That notion is a marketing gimmick.

The effects of aging often result in a more sedentary lifestyle. That alone invites accelerated, premature aging. There are several "biomarkers" of aging that can be combatted and reversed that are not so much biomarkers of aging per se, but of the sedentary lifestyles that result as consequences of aging. Many of these effects fall under the umbrella of "sarcopenia" but regular exercise, especially resistance training can improve or even reverse these effects that are considered compatible with aging - These biomarkers that represent health and well-being typically get worse as people age. Typical aging, when it is just allowed to happen and expected, looks something like this:

Effects considered to be due to aging but ones that can be improved with improved lifestyle choices:

- Tissue atrophy from disuse; in other words loss of lean mass which leads to
- Diminished strength
- Metabolic slowdown and weakened metabolic function
- Body fat increases
- Reduced and Diminished Aerobic capacity
- Blood pressure issues
- Blood-sugar balance and tolerance issues
- Bad cholesterol profiles
- Bone density problems
- Problems with body temperature regulation (a lot to do with diminished metabolism as well)

Muscle Mass: The average North American loses between five and 10 lbs of muscle mass each decade after the late 20s. Loss of muscle mass accelerates after age 45 if nothing is done about it in terms of regular exercise.

Strength: As we age, motor units deteriorate, making us weaker. Between the ages of 30 and 70, a person loses substantially greater percentage of motor unit ability each decade if nothing is done about it, as in regular exercise.

Metabolism: "normal" resting metabolic rate declines about two to five percent per decade after age 20, if nothing is done about it in terms of regular exercise.

Body fat: Between the ages of 20 and 65, the average person doubles his or her ratio of fat to muscle. This is one of the major effects of sarcopenia and a combination of all these above factors. This effect becomes more pronounced without proper diet and exercise.

Aerobic capacity: As the body ages, the ability to efficiently utilize oxygen declines substantially to as much as 40% by age 65, if nothing is done about it in terms of exercise.

Blood Sugar balance and tolerance: The body's ability to efficiently and properly use glucose (in other words glucose metabolism) declines with age, increasing the risk of Type 2 diabetes, especially proper diet and exercise.

Cholesterol/HDL levels: Healthy cholesterol profiles can diminish with age if nothing is done about it in terms of diet and exercise

Bone Density: Increased loss of calcium from bones happens with aging, making your skeletal system much weaker, if nothing is done about it in terms of diet and exercise. And this can lead to you feeling weaker as well.

Body Temperature Regulation: This tends to decline with age, especially if nothing is done about it in terms of exercise. This is why so many people are always "cold" as they age. And you can become more susceptible to both hot and cold weather influences.

These effects of aging are most often collateral effects of a sedentary lifestyle, they just become more consequential as we age if we do nothing about them. This is why I wrote, "...if nothing is done" beside so many of the above points. If you look at all these above biomarkers, you can imagine various combinations of them would make someone "feel" old as well. Feeling old makes it even more difficult to do something about it, since that "something" involves exercise.

Client Sam

I had a client named Sam who joined with me when he was around age 43. He might as well have been 70. Sam had Type 2 diabetes, a lot of chronic joint pain. He was overweight. Exercise scared him because of his diabetes and joint pain. As it turned out, his sedentary job and sedentary lifestyle, not his age, was the real problem. But it took me a long time to convince him of this.

I gently introduced Sam to easy but regular

exercise. I didn't force it on him. Eventually I coached him into liking it. A little progress can be very motivating and Sam became motivated to take the next steps himself. I got Sam on a healthy whole food diet plan with lots of healthy carbs, which he had previously been avoiding. In just over a year Sam was off his diabetes meds and although the joint pain persisted, it no longer proved debilitating, nor prevented him from exercising. The healthy whole foods diet and exercise changed his life.

Sam's story is not unique to my Coaching history. I have had many clients in the past who were able to get off of various medications, simply by following a sound diet strategy and doing a reasonable amount of exercise. The body responds to the conditions imposed on it. Not exercising at all is an intolerable condition to impose on a body, at any age, but it's especially problematic after age 50.

Similarly I have had other clients with hypertension who had somehow got the mistaken idea that this condition meant exercise was dangerous and risky for them, which is of course untrue. With proper diet strategy in place, and moderate exercise, they were able to get off their blood pressure meds and now have normal blood pressure.

In a couple of those cases, the only big change we made in diet strategy was eliminating red meat. First we eliminated it completely for six weeks. Then we just limited red meat to once per week and special occasions. Sometimes it's the smallest of differences combined together that have the biggest results and impact on health.

My goal with such clients is not to get them off these medications. That is for their doctors to decide. I just Coach them so that we improve their health incrementally.

Tufts University researchers Evans and Rosenberg (1992) discovered that all these biomarkers of health could actually be reversed or improved in older people. They immediately began promoting the benefits of exercise—specifically the importance of increasing muscle mass and strength—because these have direct and indirect healthy corollary effects on metabolism.

Since this research, study after study has illustrated that muscle is much more responsible for the body's overall vigor, verve, and vitality than most people realize. As we get older, exercise should be more about tissue "building" and all the beneficial metabolic and its biochemical effects. These are effects that are difficult to measure because they don't lend to measurements per se, and they improve over the long-term timeframe beyond how most research studies of this type are formulated. A classic mistake fitness experts still make is in thinking that exercise is about calorie "burning." The second exercise myth that persists is that exercise should be about "cardiovascular" work, as in "aerobic."

The long and the short of it is that exercising to build muscle and strength can significantly rejuvenate whole body physiology, especially as we age. And this is an additive holistic effect where "the whole is greater than the sum of its parts." As a Coach in the fitness industry this message that has been around since the early 90s is still not getting through to people age 50 and over. People still seem to be wrapped up in "cardio" as their only measure of health or fitness—and similarly they are too focused on burning calories, instead of being rightfully focused on building and keeping muscle and strength.

In one Tuft's University experiment, 12 men between the ages of 60 and 72 did weight training sessions three times per week for three months under supervision. At the conclusion of the three-month period, the subjects' strength had increased substantially. Furthermore, weight training protocols for test subjects over 95 years of age, although less intense variations, proved to be equally successful. This demonstrated once again that the body responds to the conditions imposed on it. Weight-training subjects the body to positive conditions, contributing to overall health and wellness. Being sedentary, on the other hand, invites premature, accelerated aging, and illness.

The Tufts researchers noted that subjects who undertook this form of exercise reported feeling much younger and better about themselves than they had in years. This is yet another example where biology influences mental health and well-being as well.

The conclusion is that the same exercise regimens that build muscle tend to have a holistic effect on overall health. The typical metabolic declines of old age can definitely be slowed down, halted, and even somewhat reversed with this kind of "bodybuilding" training protocol (altered to suit older individuals of course). Although all kinds of physical fitness regimens are generally linked to improved well-being, muscle building programs have proven to be the most beneficial kind of physical fitness training, in the face of the pop-culture bias against it. All of the above research conclusions support my own personal bias toward traditional body part/bodybuilding training being the best form of training for people over 50, especially in terms of combatting the usual effects of aging, or stopping the invitation toward premature, accelerated aging.

Earlier in this project I discussed the concept of "biological age." You can find many formulas for calculating biological age with a quick Google Search. What I want to point out here is significant.

In the formula I used myself, part of the calculation for biological age correctly asked the specific question, "how many times per week do you strength train." It didn't ask how many times per week do you exercise, or how much cardio do you do. It specifically asked how many times per week do you "strength train/resistance train." This shows that, to researchers who specialize in studying aging, the type of exercise regimens that keep you youthful are the resistance training/strength training workouts.

An exercise regimen after age 50 needs to soundly follow the principles of exercise physiology. This has to be balanced with recovery needs as well, no question. In any key area of life, balance is the key. So for working out with weights after age 50, moderate intensity, regular consistency, shorter duration workouts, rest and recovery are what define this balance. While the specifics of working out can vary from person to person, the above elements for an exercise regimen are what spell out balance after age 50. *Too much or too little exercise can both be issues, and training to exhaustion after age 50 can also invite accelerated, premature aging.*

To age well, and improve well-being, exercise does not have to be incredibly intense and exhausting; it just has to be a lifestyle. More and more studies are showing that even modest, consistent exercise will improve health and well-being. Someone who merely walks six days per week has a mortality rate as low as someone who runs 30 to 40 miles per week. (Institute for Aerobics Research, 1998)

After age 50, a body in balance in balance is characterized by these physiological signs:

- Strong immune system
- Balanced body rhythms and functions, such as like hunger, appetite, sleep, digestion, elimination, physical coordination, mental alertness, physical verve and vitality, sexual interest
- General enthusiasm
- A sense of spirituality

- Exhilarating and/or calming and peaceful experiences

Contrarily, combinations of these following physiological signs point to a lack of balance, creating a hindrance to aging well:

- Eczema or psoriasis (the skin is the largest organ in the body)
- Weight issues (both over- and underweight)
- Overall physical weakness (sarcopenia)
- General and/or sexual apathy
- Constipation
- General aches and pains
- Type 2 diabetes
- Always catching colds, the flu; getting constant infections of some kind
- Irregular heartbeat of any kind
- Weak kidneys and/or bladder incontinence

- Intolerance to cold weather or really hot weather
- Recurring, late-onset ADHD
- Intolerance to stress
- Worrying when there's nothing to worry about
- General restlessness, fatigue, insomnia, depression or anxiety

These negative conditions and obstructions to aging well tend to be far more prominent in people who are sedentary and inactive than they are in people who are active and exercise regularly. The question for you to ponder is how many of these above points apply to you. They have an additive effect: the more of these points that apply to you, the more out of balance you are in your triangle of awareness, and the less likely it is that you are aging well, and the more likely it is that your current lifestyle is inviting accelerated, premature aging.

* * *

You should expect more than purely physical benefits from an exercise regimen after 50, benefits like mental, emotional, and spiritual health. If your only goal for exercise is burning calories or losing weight, you're cheating yourself.

For me, training (exercise) has also been a vehicle for personal self-connection. This deep connection has intensified as I age. Now, in my mid-fifties, what I cherish most in my own training is the private, unmitigated early morning workouts. They are silent, undistracted and consistent. No compromise. No competition. No comparing myself with someone else.

Each day I value the ability to work out. That appreciation keeps me from ever taking it for granted. Working out after age 50 can be a mode of self-connection and mental restoration on a whole new plane. My book *Physique After 50* goes into greater depth of the proper exercise programming topic, if you want to investigate this on a deeper level.

Conclusion

"We've put more effort into helping folks reach old age than into helping them enjoy it."

- Frank A. Clark

Aging well is a choice.

This whole project has been about how to live better longer, how to embrace and enjoy our transition into our elder years.

You probably have a personal example or two where people with healthy lifestyles got diseases and they died relatively young. I heard of two examples the week I penned this chapter: an otherwise healthy 62-year-old man was told he has terminal cancer with only a few weeks remaining, and a former client diagnosed with early onset Alzheimer's. She's s only in her early fifties and in a long-term care facility.

After examples like these, it would be easy to question why bother with all these lifestyle considerations, when the risk of diseases and death increase substantially as we age out of our forties. It's a fair question, but also reflects wanton passivity. To me, examples like these only serve to remind just how precious it all is and that we should never take it for granted. I argue that we should consider all the ways to take better care of ourselves, taking none of our time for granted as we all likely did in our youth.

We should embrace higher expectations of what aging can bring with it; and jettison the notion that aging is about physical and mental decline. Aging shouldn't be about pining over a lost youth. It can be about finding something even more valuable. Aging should never be resented. A negative mindset over something you cannot change makes no sense. You can perceive longevity as a goal, as a gift or as an achievement, or all three. But 'qualitative' longevity only comes to those of us with high enough expectations of ourselves to reach for it. You can't give up on life or on yourself. I see and know so many people my age who have. They may not think they have given up on life but their lifestyles say otherwise. It's a pathetic thing to witness. And it is reflected in their quality of life as well.

You have three choices of how you live:

1. You can do nothing and be further behind next year than you already are.
2. You can just keep doing what you are doing now, and stay stagnant and therefore by next year you will still be behind as a matter of time drain and stagnation.
3. You can choose to better yourself.

Time passes, regardless. Are you just going to let it sweep you along, or are you going to invest yourself in it? Time becomes a more valuable commodity as you age. Today is the time to go beyond pondering a course of action. The time for action is today, for doing, growing, and for getting more use out of the time you have. Longevity after all has to be more than a goal. It should be a level of quality of experience and existence. It's an attitude toward how you live right now and today.

We've been socialized to expect far too little of aging, in mind, body, and especially spirit. But like other phases of life, aging holds just as much potential for improvement if you open your mind to the possibilities. This is the difference between having "golden years" and instead experiencing "a platinum club existence" and being age-tastic!

Deepak Chopra said, "People don't grow old; when they stop growing, they become old."

The fact is you can age in a way where you maintain youthfulness without necessary growing old, albeit a different kind and quality of youthfulness. Your life is only going to feel and be as free and liberated and invigorating as your perception of it allows. And this is especially true once the realities of aging can no longer be ignored; usually from age 50 onward.

My made-up word "age-tastic" means aging well by taking control of your life, not allowing your it to be set to "default," passively sitting by and watching age happen to you. Being age-tastic is about not taking things for granted, being introspective but in a self-supporting way. Being age-tastic is about knowing what life balance is and living in it well. Being age-tastic is about living from a place of wholeness, what I'll refer to as "the triangle of awareness"—meaning mental, emotional, and physical well-being connected and mutually supportive. Mastery of self is the path to *well-being* and *being well* at any age.

As we age beyond 50, we are offered greater freedoms and liberties than at any other time in our lives. It becomes a time to actively work on self-mastery, making it an expressive illustration for how we choose to age and live our lives by setting a higher standard for ourselves. No well-intended thought can make you age better or improve your life if it is not put into a wellness of action. A reverence and deep gratitude for the gift of a longer life lays the foundation for living better as you age.

Aging doesn't need to be feared, perceived with negative thoughts and trepidation. All your years can be vehicles for your fulfillment. The expression used to be "Life begins at 40." I say, "Life begins to awaken at 50." Life can deepen in rich experience as you age, but you have to be present. You have to want to shake hands with life and partner with it.

Remember "belief creates biology." The way you view yourself can become a self-fulfilling prophecy. If you expect to be less useful, less attractive, less energetic, less productive, and less important as you age, you probably will be.

> *"None are so old as those who have outlived enthusiasm."*
>
> *- Henry David Thoreau*

Let go of fear of death and instead embrace an enjoyment of the gift of life. Value the present moment always. Check yourself; if you catch yourself in "stinkin' thinkin'" about your own aging, remind yourself that these thoughts are devaluing the moment. To value the present means to live in it, and act within it. You will find this truth to be self-reinforcing for the rest of your years. Remember, well-being is a reflection of well-doing.

Live Inside-Out

Find and explore an inner life. Peace and calm live there. Exploit them to your own advantage. Peace of mind, contentment, and joy are paths to follow, not simply goals to have. You must choose to evolve to challenge the entropy associated with age. This is about going beyond an external battle with chronological age. You must embrace it internally, and accept the transformative experience that it is. To live with grander peace of mind as you age takes perception and perspective. It requires going inward and living from the inside out, raising your level of personal awareness regardless of what is going on around you. You will find that what is going on around you will always be less important than what is going on within you. When you learn to truly live from the inside-out, what goes on within you influences what goes on around you, more than vice versa.

Practice insight and intuition. These make you far more proactive than reactive. Learn to trust and listen to your inner voice. Know that solitude delivers peace of mind and calm self-connecting energy.

Your inner life must be enjoyable to you in order for your outer life to be. Nurture constructive, productive, positive emotions. Process and express these emotions, instead of trying to avoid or suppress negative ones. Think of your emotional fitness as a garden. You should aim to grow flowers of wellness and weed out negative emotions that interfere. You can't do that by repressing or suppressing your unwanted emotions or just trying to ignore them and pretend they aren't there. When you do that, you estrange yourself from all of your emotions and then you can't enjoy and enrich yourself from the good ones.

You have to be intelligent enough to know that almost every thought has some kind of emotion attached to it. Your emotional fitness involves experiencing an inner and satisfying fullness of self-connection, bringing an inner strength if you allow it. To ignore or suppress emotions simply isn't healthy. Doing so has greater consequences as we age. You can't grow and cultivate a healthy emotional garden if you simply ignore "weeds" that crop up. Do the healthy weeding.

Repeating unconscious habits reinforces behavior patterns, regardless of whether they are productive or destructive. Conscious awareness and behavior will create new, better lifestyle patterns that can transform age 50 and beyond into your new "Wonder Years" and to being "age-tastic." Self-investigation and introspection are essential.

Intuition, insight, introspective self-regard, and proper perspective about this transitional phase of your life—these all have a lot to do with self-respect. Self-respect gets you to become soul-trusting and self-assured, even enthusiastic. So, engage in activities and relationships that encourage self-respect.

* * *

A Few Closing Thoughts about the Body

You lose a delicate quality of vitality when you overeat, under-sleep, don't play enough, don't have enough stimulating relationships, don't have enough good sex (yes, I said it), or spending day after day in an unfulfilling occupation. This is true at any age, but as your body's physiology becomes less resilient, the negative health ramifications of these missteps become more consequential.

Your body needs regular periods of relaxation and rejuvenation through downtime. Downtime— just doing nothing— rejuvenates after being busy and occupied. Taken too far, downtime is nothing more than laziness and being sedentary. Yin and Yang – balance is the word that should center you as you age. A delicate balance in lifestyle respects the body and doesn't take it for granted.

Avoid fad diets or pop-culture diet cults. This means there's no need for fasting, cleanses, or depriving yourself of any macronutrient food group, as long as the majority of your food intake comes from healthy whole, unprocessed foods.

Be completely in tune with your rhythms. You may have to go out of your way to create a self-nurturing and youth-sustaining lifestyle. This balanced, constructive rhythm seems to be the main thing that has been lost in the modern digital era. The flow of your days and weeks needs to be something that recharges you. To age well, your day to day life should have a certain flow and rhythm that only needs to make sense to you. For example, I get up at 4:00 a.m. every day. This doesn't make sense to a lot of people. But this is me connecting fully to my own rhythm.

A word of caution: you can never fully and wholly invest in this rhythm if you are always surfing social media. As much as we are all inter-connected, we must focus on being healthily inner-connected, first and foremost. (I do not mean that you should not care about or for others.) This means avoiding too much useless, garbage-in-garbage-out mental stimulus. Instead, seek out ways to positively, purposefully, and constructively engage your mind. Reading is the best way to do this. Reading is to the mind what exercise is to the body, so remember this. But there are thousands of other ways to constructively and productively engage your mind. Find a hobby, devote yourself to it, and it will give right back to you in ways that will keep you youthful and spirited.

Laugh and play. George Bernard Shaw said, "We don't stop playing because we get old; we get old because we stop playing."

Take an interest in cultural or world events and form an opinion. It keeps your mind engaged and active and productive.

Converse with others and as importantly, converse with yourself.

I see these new transitional years of my life as a gift. I aim to give back to these years as much as I can. Maybe this is part of the secret to aging well and living age-tastically. It makes me so incredibly grateful to live in this era of ease and convenience and abundance and longer life spans, when I think that if I was born a century ago, my life would already be over. But I must not just be the recipient of these gifts. I must give back to them and give back to life as well.

You don't have to "get old." You can choose to become "age-tastic." I hope you do, and I hope this project helps!

Final Thoughts

Concrete Tips to Becoming Age-tastic!

My recommendations for experiencing a "Platinum Club" aging experience

The body thrives on regular routine. This is even truer as we pass 50. Here are some more recommendations that can improve your quality of life, and prevent you from unwittingly inviting accelerated, premature aging.

Establish regular sleep and wake times, regular pre-sleep hygiene habits, regular meal times, and if possible a regular work schedule.

Unplug more than once per day, preferably one whole day every week or two.

Take regular vacations.

Always eat breakfast.

Get outside for some minimum time period per day, as regularly as possible.

Read. Not social media or other garbage content. Read something of substance in an area of interest.

Look inside. Self-assess. As Jung put it, "Who looks outside, dreams—who looks inside, awakens." Age 50+ is a great time for your own personal true and authentic awakening.

Nourish your emotions with self-supporting thoughts. Remind yourself that emotions make good guides, but terrible masters.

Self-direct your thoughts. If you don't like a current line of thinking, "Change the channel."

Avoid anything with the prefix "over," such as overworked, overburdened, over-scheduled, overly stressed, overly worried, overexertion, overexcitement or overstimulated.

Make time every day for simple rest and

rejuvenation. Take a break. Energy has to be recharged or it simply runs out.

Find the equal balance between contributing to your day, and enjoying it.

Find stability in as many things as you can: Your work, your relationships, your finances. If any of these things isn't working, make a change.

Find a space and place to invite calm peaceful energy. Just "be" with yourself for a while every day.

Find a self-connecting activity that gives you peace and calm, that nurtures and invigorates you at the same time. For me, this is reading, movies and my working out. For others it may be golf, hiking, gardening, bird-watching, coin collecting, cooking, or camping. It doesn't matter what "it" is, as long as it is self-connecting for you.

Remember small positive habits add up.

The essence of all of this is that well-doing leads to well-being. Create cheerful conditions for yourself and find a way to enjoy a quiet solitude on a regular basis. Embrace the profound wisdom of Philippians

4:8. "Finally, brothers and sisters, whatever is true, whatever is noble, whatever is right, whatever is pure, whatever is lovely, whatever is admirable—if anything is excellent or praiseworthy—think about such things." Write this down somewhere and use it to self-investigate your thinking at any given time. Chances are if you are feeling negative in a given moment it's because you are thinking negatively and unclearly. This verse is a way to get you into the habit of self-directed constructive and productive thought.

Appendix

Noteworthy Age-tastic Quotes

I thought I would share a few memorable quotes on graceful, age-tastic aging, many from people with noteworthy achievements later in life.

Forty is the old age of youth; fifty the youth of old age.

- Victor Hugo

Age is no barrier. It's a limitation you put on your mind.

- Jackie Joyner-Kersee

How old would you be if you didn't know how old you are?

- Satchel Paige

People tell me I look good these days. I look good because I feel good. I know people who are older than I am who are twenty-five... It's all about attitude. To me, age is just a number.

- Rita Moreno

I think that, for all of us, as we grow older, we must discipline ourselves to continue expanding, broadening, learning, keeping our minds active and open.

— Clint Eastwood

One thing that can make us old fast is thinking that we are getting old.

— Robert P. Lockwood
(A Guy's Guide to the Good Life)

There is a fountain of youth: it is your mind, your talents, the creativity you bring to your life and the lives of people you love. When you learn to tap this source, you will truly have defeated age.

— Sophia Loren

This is a youth-oriented society, and the joke is

on them because youth is a disease from which we all recover.

- Dorothy Fuldheim

You are as young as your faith, as old as your doubt; as young as your self-confidence, as old as your fear as young as your hope, as old as your despair.

- Douglas MacArthur

Nobody grows old by merely living a number of years. People grow old only by deserting their ideals. Years may wrinkle the skin, but to give up interest wrinkles the soul.

- Douglas MacArthur

It's sad to grow old, but nice to ripen.

- Brigitte Bardot

I look forward to being older, when what you look like becomes less and less an issue and what you are is the point.

- Susan Sarandon

Anyone who stops learning is old, whether this happens at twenty or eight. Anyone who keeps on learning not only remains young, but becomes constantly more valuable regardless of physical capacity.

- Harvey Ullman

Age is of no importance unless you are a cheese.

- Billie Burke

Age is an issue of mind over matter. If you don't mind, it doesn't matter.

- Mark Twain

As I approve of a youth that has something of the old man in him, so I am no less pleased with an old man that has something of the youth. He that follows this rule may be old in body, but can never be so in mind.

- Cicero

I have enjoyed greatly the second blooming that comes when you finish the life of the emotions and of personal relations; and suddenly find—at the age of fifty, say—that a whole new life has opened before you, filled with things you can think about, study, or read about...It is as if a fresh sap of ideas and thoughts was rising in you.

- Agatha Christie

I'm not interested in age. People who tell me their age are silly. You're as old as you feel.

- Elizabeth Arden

It takes a long time to become young.

- Pablo Picasso

The more sand [that] has escaped from the hourglass of our life, the clearer we should see through it.

- Jean-Paul Sartre

Youth is the gift of nature, but age is a work of art.

- Stanislaw Lec

Belief creates biology.

- Norman Cousins

Our bodies are our gardens, to the which our wills are the gardeners.

- Shakespeare, from Othello

When it comes to staying young, a mind-lift beats a face-lift any day.

- Marty Bucella

I live in that solitude which is painful in youth, but delicious in the years of maturity.

- Albert Einstein

THANK YOU

I would like to take a moment and say *thank you* for purchasing this book. And a second *thank you* for reading all the way to the end.

There are plenty of books now about how to deal with aging — not to mention endless opinions and articles about it on the Internet — but you chose this one, took the time to read it, and that means a lot.

If you have a moment, I would love it if you could leave the book a review on Amazon. Feedback helps me improve. And if you loved the book, I would *love* to hear about that as well!

A Free Gift

As a thank you for getting this book, you can download the Abel Starter Set, including *The Mindset of Achievement* and *Intro to Metabolic Enhancement Training (MET)* (yes, the entire books) completely free.

The Mindset of Achievement is about reaching goals and sustaining them and building on them. If you've ever achieved something (e.g. weight loss) only to find you couldn't sustain the success, this book is for you. It has chapters on habits & routines, motivation, getting out of "ruts," fear of failure, mastery and much more.

Intro to Metabolic Enhancement Training (MET) explains the methodology behind this unique metabolic training program, and includes two full 4-day programs.

Just go to **scottabelfitness.com/starter** to get your copies from the homepage.

Other Works

by Scott Abel

Please visit scottabelfitness.com/ebooks

Nutrition, Diet and Weight Loss

The Anti-Diet Approach

Beyond Metabolism

The Cycle Diet

Metabolic Damage

Permanent Weight Loss

Understanding Metabolism

Training

The Abel Approach

Better Abs, Stronger Core

The Busy Woman's Train-at-Home Program

The Hardgainer Solution

How to Train for a Better Physique

The MET Workshop Workbook

Intro to Metabolic Enhancement Training (or 'MET')

The Slingshot Program

Your First Proper 6-Day Bodybuilding Training Program

Mindset and More

How to Be An Insanely Good Fitness Coach

The Mindset of Achievement

Zen Fitness, Tao Health

© Copyright Scott Abel

Endnotes

[1] Quoted in Dean, Jeremy. "When These Muscles Are Fitter Your Brain Is Also Fitter." *PsyBlog*. 29 Nov. 2015. Web. <http://www.spring.org.uk/2015/11/when-these-muscles-are-fitter-your-brain-is-also-fitter.php>

[2] Steves, Claire J et al. "Kicking Back Cognitive Ageing: Leg Power Predicts Cognitive Ageing After Ten Years in Older Female Twins." *Gerontology* 62.2 (2016): 138–149. Web. <http://www.karger.com/?doi=10.1159/000441029>

[3] A 2011 review of the literature on the subject, looking at 16 unrelated studies, found that a 1-standard deviation advantage in cognitive test scores was associated with a 24% lower risk of death when subjects were followed up with between 17 and 69 years later. See Calvin, C M et al. "Intelligence in Youth and All-Cause-Mortality: Systematic Review with Meta-Analysis." *International Journal of Epidemiology* 40.3 (2011):

626-644.

4   See Belloc, Nedra B, and Lester Breslow. "Relationship of Physical Health Status and Health Practices." *Preventative Medicine* 1.2 (1972): 409-421. Print. (Their research has been very heavily cited and you can find out about it with a quick Google search.)

5   See Marlatt, G A, and J L Kristeller. "Mindfulness and Meditation." *Integrating Spirituality Into Treatment*. Ed. W R Miller. Washington, DC: American Psychologiclal Association, 1999. I originally found the quotation in a review of mindfulness training by Ruth Baer. See Baer, R A. "Mindfulness Training as a Clinical Intervention: a Conceptual and Empirical Review." *Clinical Psychology: Science and Practice* 10.2 (2003): 125-143.

Printed in Great Britain
by Amazon